Let It Flow:

Blood Flow Is the True Fountain of Youth

Preface

Introduction

Chapter 1: Understanding Our Circulation

Key Players
Blood Flow
Hardening of the Arteries and Plaque Buildup
Problems Can Start Early in Life
A Surgeon's Perspective
Athletes
Emergencies

Chapter 2: How Our Circulation Impacts the Body

Skin
Heart
Liver
Mental Health
Vision
Hair
Sexual Function
Strong Muscles

Chapter 3: Factors That Influence Our Circulation

Inflammation
Cholesterol
Sugar
Smoking
Processed Food
Stress

Chapter 4: Diseases of Our Circulation

High Blood Pressure
Diabetes
Obesity
Heart Disease

Stroke
Metabolic Syndrome
Alzheimer's Disease
Cancer

Chapter 5: Linking Aging to Our Circulation

The Aging Process
Chronological Versus Biological Aging
Premature Aging
Blue Zone
Research on Aging
Aging Blood Vessels

Chapter 6: Unleashing the Power of Our Circulation

Eat Right
Eat Less
Move More
Be Better Informed
Metformin

Preface

I was maybe five when my parents sent my two brothers and me to the countryside outside our home city of Seoul, Korea, to live with our grandparents. My parents, promising to send for us when they were financially stable, went to the suburbs of New York seeking the American Dream. While my grandparents ran a small malt liquor factory, we boys went to school, learned English, and ran around the fields and barns of local farmers, most of whom lived in mud huts with grass-thatched roofs. We raised chickens and pigs out back. How often I'd run out to get a newly laid egg from under a chicken, poke a hole in the top and bottom, and suck out the yolk and white. Or watch as my grandmother boiled it and added it to our soup. But what I remember most is the fresh fruits and vegetables we'd eat from the fields and stand along the dirt roads—the juicy apples, lush pink watermelon, and bright-red strawberries; an occasional roasted green grasshopper; the Chinese cabbage, radish, and squash my grandmother would shred up for kimchi; the pumpkins we'd pick up from the Ahns' house; the pears ripe and ready on the tree.

A simple life, for sure, which included walking everywhere since we, like most people in rural Korea, didn't have cars or bikes. Even the men who delivered kegs from the malt liquor factory wheeled around on bicycles.

Occasionally, we'd stop at the cart vendors selling *ppopgi*, melted sugar sprinkled with baking soda. Using technique, timing, and patience, the vendor would create before our eyes a sweet, melt-in-your mouth, light snack in the shape of a bird, fish, star, or figurine. If we could eat all the candy base around the design without cracking it, we'd get an extra ppopgi. Sugar as sport!

After a few years, we finally made our way, via JFK airport, to a suburban town sixty miles outside of New York City. The big surprise our parents had for us were bicycles. We rode *everywhere*—to our newfound friends' houses and to the post office. Later, after working as a golf caddy, I made enough money to buy myself a ten-speed bike. My world expanded; now I could bike to the mall or the beach or local coin and stamp shops in the surrounding towns. If I wasn't studying, working, or lifting the weights I'd bought hoping to get a spot on the school football team, I was on that bike.

[i]

Assimilation being key to the success of an immigrant family like ours, we learned English quickly and started eating American foods, which meant hamburgers, hot dogs, mac and cheese, and Coca-Cola, and having family nights out at Kentucky Fried Chicken and McDonald's. The nights we'd eat traditional Korean food, we'd feast on meat and tofu soup, rice and a medley of marinated vegetables.

At some point, my father developed diabetes as a result of a poor diet and excessive alcohol consumption. He started subscribing to *Prevention* magazine to help with the management of his disease. Not only did he then change his diet, but he also demanded that all of us children steer clear of desserts, sweets, and added sugar and eat plenty of fruits and vegetables. He had us eating whole wheat rather than white bread for breakfast. My dad became thin and always on the move, often doing all sorts of manual labor. He controlled his sugar level with diet only and no medication. He kept us all busy— putting in a septic tank, building stone walls in the yard, planting gardens and tending them, fixing our home. Working out became part of my routine, as did even trying to bulk up by eating peanut butter sandwiches.

Then came college and medical school, where I studied hard, drank excessive amounts of alcohol on occasion; ate lots of fast food, potato chips, and packaged foods; and even smoked the occasional cigarette. It didn't seem to be that different from what other twentysomethings were doing, as we were young and healthy and nearly invincible—or so we thought. Ironically, as a medical student, I thought very little about what was happening inside my own body or how I was taking care of it. I was young, in good health, and getting sick never entered my mind.

Being a doctor represented respect, prestige, financial security, and a way to make the sick feel better. I was idealistic in my beliefs about patient care, as most medical students are. My favorite course was anatomy, and during cadaver dissections, I was fascinated by how amazing the human body is. Mapping out the bones, muscles, organs, nerves, and blood vessels in anatomy lab and learning how to work with tissues revealed surgery to be my true calling. It seemed to provide immediate gratification, which I liked a lot. Treating the chronic diseases we learned in classes like pathology, pharmacology, and internal medicine didn't appeal to me because it didn't seem like patients ever really got better. On the other hand, surgeons took care of patients with immediate results—or so I thought. Nobody in medical school was talking about nutrition or exercise or prevention—it was either disease treatment or surgery.

I settled on surgery, specifically plastic surgery, and came to New York City to train. As a plastic surgeon, you have the ability to make people happier, whether by performing a facelift, a nose job, or restoring a breast after cancer. I could make them look better and feel more positive about their outward appearance. Having an appreciation for shape and symmetry gave me an edge, and I quickly found a phenomenal place in healthcare.

Life was busy; I paid little attention to what I put in my body or how much I exercised. I stopped by the gym when I could and was fairly oblivious to what I was eating and how often I ate. All of this was based on some loose notions of what I perceived as healthy.

So again, I wasn't thinking about how I or my family, friends, and patients were treating our insides because, for the most part, we all looked healthy on the outside. And if someone didn't, I could fix them with surgery. I hadn't really processed that old saying "you can't judge a book by its cover" yet.

About five years ago, a patient of mine brought in a book that linked nutrition to chronic disease and pointed out that people in several rural areas around the world who ate simply and moved out of necessity seemed to have an unusually low incidence of chronic disease. Reading it and then fervently seeking out confirming research, I thought back to my time in the Korean countryside, the simplicity of life, of the foods we ate, and the way we were always on the move. And it made me think a lot about my father's urging to bring us closer to that way of living after he was diagnosed with diabetes.

My life and surgical career have highlighted the dilemma that began from my medical school days—the most common and costly chronic disease that plagues Americans can't be reversed. But I've learned that diseases like heart disease, hypertension, cancer, diabetes, and obesity aren't just treatable; they are preventable. It's taken a lot of life experience, research, soul searching, and flashbacks to my childhood years to figure it all out. And is so often the case, the simplest solution turns out to be the best truth. Like me, you may have known the key to health at one point and then forgotten it. When I put it all together, I saw that the way we live life in America is perpetuating an unhealthy, slowed blood flow. This lifestyle is resulting in a country that spends more money on healthcare than it does on quality food. We've become accustomed to quick fixes and we keep looking for answers in a bottle or a pill or new legislation.

Years of making incisions and dissections during surgery clarified to me how important blood flow is to the health of the entire body. From a surgeon's perspective, patients with chronic disease have sluggish blood flow, darker blood and poorer tissue quality compared to healthy people. Know this: our cells, tissues, and organs need brisk, bright-red blood full of oxygen to function properly!

Connecting the dots, it became apparent to me that blood flow—the same criteria I used in determining a successful surgery or a potential outcome—was central to how we age and how chronic diseases develop and affect us. The bottom line of all that healthy eating and exercising? Protecting our blood vessels.

Anything that damages our blood vessels can lead to problems in our body. It doesn't happen randomly or just because we age—what we do, eat, drink, smoke can cause damage we won't be able to see for many years down the line. We can look good on the outside but be causing injury on the inside.

As a plastic surgeon, I thought outward appearance of patients was more essential than the inner dynamics of their bodies. Since my job often involves making people look more youthful, many see me as an antiaging expert. The truth is that plastic surgeons are no more purveyors of the fountain of youth than anti-aging researchers, cosmetics, or pharmaceutical companies. I came to realize, over time, that my patients had more power over their health and beauty than I'd ever guessed, but by not telling them how to care for the very viable fountain of youth they have inside, I wasn't living up to the Hippocratic Oath.

Introduction

Before launching into a crash course on aging and hemodynamics, I'm going to give you a gift. But the truth is, you already own it.

That's the single most important takeaway from this book: you already own the closest thing to the fountain of youth.

Truth be told, renowned researchers, pharmaceutical companies, savvy marketers, well-trained surgeons, dermatologists, physicians, personal trainers, nutritionists, and diet gurus cannot deny that you already own what is regarded as the best-known way to help keep your body healthy, your skin glowing, your hair full, your organs working, your sexuality inspired, and your vision sharp. You always have. Free and clear.

So here's my gift.

Your circulatory system holds the key to your health and youthfulness.

After years of study, surgery, consulting, researching the evidence, and living, I believe that if health is an equation with one solution, the very best evidence-based solution currently available is getting your blood to circulate all over your body—regularly and smoothly.

Flooding your cells and tissues with oxygen and nutrients + getting rid of the wastes = healthy circulation. Healthy circulation = healthy cells = health.

In your lifetime, your heart will pump about one million barrels of blood through the body to your organs. Right now, your heart is circulating about six quarts of blood throughout your body three times every minute—and as amazing as it sounds, your blood is traveling 12,000 miles or the equivalent of four coast-to-coast road trips across the United States every single day! If you unraveled and laid out all the arteries, veins, and capillaries of your circulatory system, you'd have to circle Earth about two and a half times.

All that is what keeps you healthy.

You can stop waiting for a better answer or handing out more money to pursue a better solution or for someone to uncover a medical fountain of youth.

The truth is that many of the surgeries, medications, exercises, and diets the experts can offer you all trace back one way or another to helping the circulatory system do its job more efficiently and effectively. Most of the research being done into antiaging right now involves blood and circulation in some way. It's that simple. Really.

I hope this is liberating. I hope this truth helps make sense of the variety of contradicting messages about how to live a healthy life—at the center of it all is circulation.

How can you best affect circulation? Pretty basically you want to move, eat well, not worry too much, and not smoke.

Knowledge is power. And with great power comes great responsibility, which is both a gift and a curse, as Spider-Man likes to say. What are *you* going to do with this power?

This book is going to give you some ideas. You'll learn truths about your body, and, in the process, I'll help you unleash the power of your circulatory system, so you can prevent diseases, slow down aging, and even avoid cancer. If you think of your circulatory system as a personal treasure, then by simply getting your blood to course through your vessels is central to health and wellness.

Let's start now.

Chapter 1: Understanding Our Circulatory System

Prominent doctors and medical historians from the University of California and Stanford University have crowned circulation as "the single most important discovery of Western medicine." That's right: English doctor William Harvey's discovery of the circulatory system in the early part of the 1600s beats out vaccinations, surgical anesthesia, diagnostic x-rays, antibiotics, and genetic engineering.

His description of circulation as a vital process that follows the rules of physics was groundbreaking. He declared that the heart's sole purpose was to pump blood. Earth-shattering! Imagine—proving that blood flows in a circular motion, is pumped from the heart, carried from each ventricle by arteries and arterioles to tissues in *every part* of the body, and is then transported back to the heart through veins and venules, where it starts the journey all over again, continuously going around and around and around, was akin to Galileo asserting that the Earth revolved around the Sun. And as ideas that balk at tradition often are, it was at first called heresy and fraud.

It's hard to believe that the idea of blood moving in a continuous circle was such a big deal, because today it's just basic physiology. But in the 1600s, it was totally radical.

Despite the fact that Harvey had researched the mechanics of blood flow for thirteen years and performed many animal dissections, experiments with snakes, autopsies, and clinical observations, he still feared for his life from angry and jealous peers and worried that the whole of humanity would hate him.

But if Harvey is considered the father of modern physiology, then Claudius Galen, a Greek doctor to the gladiators (think of all the trauma and open wounds he must have treated) and physician to Emperor Marcus Aurelius is regarded as the founder of experimental physiology. Galen, who lived about 1,500 years earlier than Harvey and had never done a human dissection, somehow cornered the market on teachings about blood for more than fourteen centuries. When Harvey presented his discovery in his book *On the Motion of the Heart and Blood in Animals* in 1628, he was debunking the teachings of a legend whose ideas had dominated medical science for a very long time.

[1]

Galen and his over-a-millennium's worth of physician followers believed that blood was made in the liver, from food and nutrients provided by the stomach. Dissecting human corpses was taboo back in the first and second centuries, so Galen had only dissected animals. As a result, he jumped to the conclusion that some blood vessels and structures that he'd seen in animals also existed in people. (To be fair, some of what Galen observed about the skeleton, respiration, the spinal cord, the larynx, and more was correct and is still considered pretty brilliant.) He himself also disproved some long-held notions, like the ancient idea that arteries carried air instead of blood. Unfortunately, in his view, the heart was a vacuum and home of the spirit. Galen wasn't alone in this mystical thinking about the heart—the ancient Egyptians believed it was the seat of emotions and intellect, and the Chinese called it the "place where happiness lives." (If you've ever bought a Valentine's card, scratched your beloved's name in a heart onto a tree trunk, or felt the pain of a "broken" heart, you've also been mimicking these age-old notions.)

So for almost a millennium and a half, physicians had been treating sick patients based on Galen's view of blood. Unfortunately, among other things, Galen encouraged the theory of "humorism." According to Galen and the many physicians who had followed him for all those years, disease was caused by excess blood that had gone bad from lying stagnant too long, like the water in a pond. In his view, the only way to get rid of what doctors considered "excess or weakened blood" was to sweat, urinate, or bleed it out. Bloodletting was the preferred cure, and it was generally prescribed by a doctor but carried out by a barber-surgeon. You know those red-and-white and sometimes blue barber poles outside barbershops? They symbolized the red blood and the white bandages (as well as blue veins if the blue was used).

And then, along came Harvey with his seventy-two-page treatise on circulation. He had studied at the University of Padua, possibly with Galileo Galilei, who was a professor there at the time. Even while he researched the circulatory system, he worked as physician to King James I and other aristocrats. He worked without a microscope and often accused of quackery by his colleagues. Sometimes he even doubted himself, saying, "The heart's motion is only to be comprehended by God."

[2]

Nevertheless, he pressed on, measuring the volume of a human's left ventricle and calculating that the amount of blood passing through the heart of a person in thirty minutes is more than the amount of blood contained in their entire body. He went on to show that the blood in the arteries and veins was *not* of the same origin, was *not* manufactured from food in the liver or air in the lungs; that tissues did *not* consume blood; and that blood was *not* air but liquid. Perhaps most importantly, he strongly insisted that the circulatory system was a closed circuit.

It took many years for physicians to accept the truth of his theory and change their ways, including ending the barbaric practice of bloodletting. And of course, Harvey didn't answer all the questions. The exact link between arteries and veins, for example, eluded him. It wasn't until thirty years later, when Italian biologist and physician Marcello Malpighi, using a newly improved microscope, looked at the fine structure of the lung tissue through a microscope and saw tiny thread vessels that connected arteries to veins, that the theory of a closed system for blood pumping from the heart to the tissues and back was proven.

Thank Harvey and Malpighi for confirming that your blood travels around your body in a loop and is pumped by the heart. Whatever is in your blood goes everywhere, touches every tissue, and runs through your heart 24-7. Or at least it's supposed to if everything is working properly.

But why? Well, not Galen nor Harvey nor Malpighi could answer that—but we can. The heart and blood vessels deliver oxygen, nutrients, immune cells, and hormones to every cell in the body. Without blood, organs will fail. Imagine the chaos that can cause:

Early aging. Disease. Death.

Key Players

To be firing on all pistons, you need the oxygen in your blood to combust with the carbohydrates, proteins, and fats in the food you eat—a process called *respiration*, which happens in the mitochondria (cell's powerhouse) of each of the thirty-seven trillion cells in your body.

It is not unlike what goes on inside a car engine: air is sucked into the cylinders where fuel and oxygen are mixed into a highly combustible state and ignited by a spark plug, which causes a controlled explosion. This explosion in turn drives a piston. The piston transfers energy to the crankshaft allowing the car to move.

In your body, oxygen and nutrients are utilized to produce energy, and carbon dioxide and waste products are released into the blood. This energy is then used to drive all the cellular processes necessary for us to live. Without respiration, you won't have energy, and eventually, you'll die—or at least the cells deprived of it will die.

Blood is made up of red blood cells, white blood cells, platelets, and plasma. The red blood cells carry oxygen, which is vital in creating the energy in your body. White blood cells fight off foreign invaders and infectious diseases that can destroy your cells. Platelets help your blood to clot when necessary, so you won't lose too much of it when injured, for instance. Plasma is the yellowish liquid in the blood that carries nutrients, hormones, and proteins.

Together, they make up blood—the only thing in your body that truly interacts and sends messages everywhere. I like to think of it as our bodies' information superhighways in that regard.

Blood touches *everything*, and it is involved in every aspect of your life—eating, sleeping, breathing, exercising, thinking, sex, aging, appearance, and pretty much any illness, addiction, or disease you'll suffer. But you won't necessarily know when problems with your circulatory system start.

And just like on a highway, even a tiny accident can jam up traffic or turn a four-lane highway into a one-lane road.

At the beginning of this journey is the heart, the hardest-working organ in your body and the force that energizes the players. Its muscles never stop contracting, pumping relentlessly every minute of every day for as many years as you live. Relatively simple and only the size of a man's clenched fist, it weighs less than a pound but can pump about two to three ounces of blood with every beat. While the total amount of blood in your body is about five liters (or five quarts), your heart is pumping 280 liters every single hour. Without the thrust provided by the heart's contractions, blood would pool in the lowest points of the body, unable to make the return trip to the heart. While your heart pumps out blood, it also needs the oxygen and nutrients to be delivered to itself. This is where the vital components of the circulatory system come in.

[4]

Let's start with the arteries—they carry blood away from the heart. Veins bring it back to the heart. They follow two routes: Pulmonary Road and Systemic Road.

Travel on Pulmonary Road is straightforward: this short route takes blood through the lungs, to pick up oxygen and returns to the heart before the major journey on the Systemic Road begins.

Along Systemic Road, oxygen and nutrient-rich blood are transported out of the heart to *all* the organs, tissues, and cells, which happens about seventy times per minute. If Systemic Road gets blocked or slowed in any way, be assured that some tissues somewhere in your body will suffer. Traveling on Systemic Road, there's a main artery that branches into smaller arteries and arterioles, which are simply vascular highways that provide a pathway for your blood. The arteries continue to branch into ever-smaller vessels, which connect to the tiny capillaries, those elusive vessels that Harvey couldn't identify and Malpighi eventually discovered.

It is through the thin walls of the capillaries that the circulatory system's most important swap—the exchange of oxygen and nutrients for carbon dioxide and waste—happens. Capillaries are packed together in capillary beds. If you could see them they would appear as endless back alleys that lead to each and every tissue and cell in your body. Since there are so many of them, and their diameters are so narrow, blood travels very slowly through these capillary beds. That slow pace is what makes them the perfect place to exchange gases, nutrients, hormones, and wastes between blood and cells. A capillary has the same diameter as a red blood cell and collectively, they cover about a thousand square miles in your body!

On any highway, traffic that flows along smoothly, without a jam or delay, is always preferred. To make that more likely, the vast network of arteries, veins, and capillaries are all designed with a smooth-surfaced, inner sheath of microscopic cells called endothelial cells, which provide an even surface to keep blood flowing smoothly. Hundreds of millions of cells—when placed end to end, they would wrap more than four times around the Earth and together are called the *endothelium*—line blood vessels from the heart down to the smallest capillary. The lining forms a thin layer between the vessel walls and the flowing blood, and serves as the boundary, or interface, by which blood signals to the rest of our body. While these

[5]

cells would weigh as much as the liver when put together, they are not even visible to the human eye. Previously written off as simply a Teflon-like lining, researchers and doctors now consider the endothelial lining essential to health and very vulnerable to injury, which can cause problems all over our body.

TIPS: Drink water. About 60 percent of our bodies, and 85 percent of our brains, is made up of water. Water is vital to our circulatory system, as even mild dehydration slows blood flow because blood becomes more viscous as it loses water. This can cause headaches, dry skin, constipation, muscle cramps, and sleepiness. Dehydration can be due to menstruation, high blood sugar, prescription meds, low-carb diets, stress, irritable bowel syndrome, exercise, pregnancy, dietary supplements, high altitudes, breastfeeding, and alcohol. As we age, our body's ability to conserve water and our sense of thirst is altered.

Drink seven to ten cups (8 ounces) of water per day to keep your blood flowing smoothly.

Make sure you're not anemic by having your blood count checked annually. If you have low red blood cell count, find the source of the anemia. Anemia will compromise oxygen supply to every cell in your body. Taking iron supplements or consuming food rich in iron like shellfish, spinach, beans, tofu, and red meats will bolster your red blood cell count.

Blood Flow

The ability of blood to get where it needs to go is crucial. Jean-Louis-Marie Poiseuille, a French physician and physiologist, was so curious about what caused differences in blood flow that, in 1839, he started experimenting with liquids in narrow tubes. Through his experiments, he formulated an equation to calculate rate of blood flow. Called Poiseuille's Law, it looks like this:

$$Flow\ rate = \pi PR^4 / 8nL$$

Basically, it says that blood flows at a rate based on its viscosity (n), the length of the blood vessel (L), the pressure in the blood vessel (P), and the radius (half the diameter) of the blood vessel (R). The diameter of the blood vessel has the greatest

[6]

influence on the blood flow, varying its size through contraction and expansion. Poiseuille showed that even a minor change in the diameter of a blood vessel could make a tremendous difference in the flow rate of oxygen-rich blood to tissue. For instance, a 50 percent reduction in the diameter of a blood vessel will decrease the flow of blood by 94 percent. On the other hand, 50 percent enlargement in the diameter of a blood vessel will increase the blood flow fivefold! That's why your blood vessels' ability to expand and contract is so critical.

Importance of Flexibility

Healthy blood vessels are elastic and dynamic and have the capacity to expand (also known as *vasodilation*) and contract (*vasoconstriction*) thanks to the smooth muscle that lies beneath the endothelium. Strong and rubber-band-like arteries can expand to handle surges of blood and then recover by returning to their original size. Being flexible allows them to change their diameter and manage blood flow with versatility, adjusting the movement of blood into and through different tissues.

Blood vessels relax or expand to allow blood to flow into organs and tissues that require more oxygen to create energy. Vasodilation can also occur when the tissue isn't getting enough nutrients, such as glucose and fats. It's essential that vessels are flexible enough to expand. Your overall health is absolutely dependent upon this quality.

Relaxed blood vessels lead to lower blood pressure. When it is cold outside, the vessels near your skin contract to keep blood away from cold skin, and the vessels deep inside your body expand to increase blood flow toward your core to preserve heat. Blood vessel expansion happens during exercise, movement, digestion, sex, and when your body experiences temperature changes.

Constriction is what your healthy vessels do to adjust blood flow, reduce excessive blood loss, and to prevent a drop in blood pressure, like when you stand up. Blood vessels constrict and blood pressure is maintained.

Here's a peek at how blood vessels change their diameter: If you looked through a microscope into the cross-section of a healthy artery, you'd see thin walls and a large *lumen*—the open space inside the blood vessel through which the blood flows. When the blood vessel expands, the lumen enlarges, allowing more blood to flow, but when it constricts, the lumen narrows, slowing the blood flow.

The arteries in your body branch into narrower, thinner-walled arterioles that are less sturdy. Arterioles are uniquely responsible for meeting the demands of the body by controlling the movement of blood into tissues and organs. In response to physical exertion, digesting a meal, or some other physiological event, our body sends signals to enlarge arterioles in one site and narrow them elsewhere. These signals that lead to vessel expansion come from different sources, such as nerve impulses, hormones, and a biological messenger that includes nitric oxide released from the endothelium to affect the smooth muscle beneath it.

During exercise, vasodilation boosts energy production and improves the removal of waste products like lactic acid and ammonia that can cause muscle fatigue or cramping. Athletes are especially conscious of their need to have flexible blood vessels that can expand and deliver more blood when needed.

Arterial stiffness is the opposite of flexibility. It is the result of repeated injuries to the blood vessel, limiting the smooth muscles (within the blood vessel) to relax and expand. When the arteries become rigid and less rubber-band-like, they can't expand to provide more blood flow, which can lead to high blood pressure and lower oxygen delivery to cells. This can occur even in young people if they suffer from obesity and sugar problems (diabetes or insulin resistance). Modern technology has given us a way to measure blood vessel stiffness by looking at pulse wave velocity (PWV). This can be done in the doctor's office.

TIPS: Foods rich in nitrates, flavonoids, and L-arginine are great nutrients to maximize nitric oxide in the blood. Nitrate-rich spinach, beets, and leaf lettuce interact with saliva to turn nitrates into nitrites and then get swallowed and digested in the stomach with gastric acid, which turns them into nitric oxide—exactly what you need to relax your blood vessel walls.

Flavonoids contribute to an increase in the production of nitric oxide in the body, which makes your blood vessels more elastic. They are found in foods such as broccoli, spinach, and kale. A recent study published in the American

Journal of Clinical Nutrition links particular flavonoids found in blueberries, blackberries, strawberries, grapes, cherries, and apples with a reduced risk of erectile dysfunction, a problem frequently caused by an inability of certain blood vessels to expand and deliver blood[1].
The amino acid L-arginine, found in red meat, chicken, fish, cheese, milk, eggs, and nuts like almonds and walnuts, is also helpful in producing nitric oxide and getting blood vessels to expand.

Hardening of the Arteries and Plaque Buildup

When blood vessels become thick *and* stiff, doctors call it *arteriosclerosis*. Colloquially, it's referred to as "hardening of the arteries."

If you add an *h* and take out the *i*, you get *atherosclerosis*, a specific type of arteriosclerosis, which refers to the buildup of fatty material and other substances *in* your artery walls (plaques), which can restrict blood flow, burst, and perhaps trigger a blood clot. This happens as the arteries harden further. As the plaque grows, it narrows the open space (*lumen*) in the artery tubes, reducing oxygen and blood flow to organs. If it blocks an artery supplying the heart or the brain, it may lead to a heart attack or a stroke and becomes a life-threatening emergency.

Even before it becomes life-threatening though, it is a complicated disease involving our body's immune system, especially inflammation—that same kind of red, swollen, painful reaction you see when you scrape your knee by falling over your shoelace and landing on the pavement. Most of the time, inflammation is a lifesaver that allows our body to fight off disease-causing bacteria, viruses, and parasites. But sometimes, our bodies go too far, creating more problems, harming us with what experts refer to as *friendly fire*.

This goes against old theories that presented atherosclerosis as a straightforward plumbing problem, like a pipe that clogs from too much gunk. In reality, researchers have learned that artery walls aren't passive; arteries aren't lifeless conduits. It's not as simple as saying that fatty goop builds up around the artery walls, and then plaque grows big enough to block off the open part of the vessel. That happens sometimes, but not in most cases. Truthfully, few of the plaque deposits that grow within vessel walls ever reach a size large enough to almost completely obstruct the opening through which the blood flows. Most heart attacks and a predominant number of strokes are caused by smaller plaques that break off and form a blood clot, which then obstructs the flow.

There's plenty of evidence that our blood vessels are full of living cells that are constantly communicating with each other and the surrounding environment. They are active participants in the development and growth of atherosclerotic deposits *within*, not *on*, the vessel walls.

Problems in our blood vessels that slow flow and limit a vessel's ability to expand and contract can begin in our younger years. The protective barrier lining our blood vessels gets injured or breached, making them vulnerable. Once a break in the *endothelium* (blood vessel lining) occurs, our body's immune system kicks in and inflammation begins. White blood cells begin to cling to the lining to stabilize the damage. Just as a skinned knee eventually turns into a scab as it heals, the body tries to patch the injured area in our blood vessel, sending in a repair crew consisting of lipids (cholesterol, triglycerides and other fats), clotting factors, and white cells— resulting in a *plaque*. What started as the body trying to repair an injury suddenly begins the process of atherosclerosis.

But when inflammation persists, the white blood cells can worsen the injury. Breaks in the lining of the endothelium allow certain lipids to penetrate the wall of the blood vessel, becoming easily oxidized by free radical making the vessels resemble a rusted metal pipe.

Remember: Artery walls aren't passive and the living cells in blood vessels communicate with each other. The oxidized lipids signal to the cells in the vessel walls to repair the damage.

Next thing you know, different kinds of *macrophages* (immune cells that engulf and remove) are arriving to digest and scavenge the lipid deposits, becoming frothy, known as *foam cells*. This growing mass further sets off body's immune response.

To keep the plaque content contained, the smooth muscle cells (remember this muscle is involved in contraction and relaxation of blood vessels) produce collagen to form a fibrous cap at the injured site. Sometimes smooth muscle itself becomes so altered by injury and inflammation that it becomes a participant, adding calcium to the developing plaque. As more plaque builds up along the blood vessel, the wall gets thick and stiff. As the hardening of the arteries progresses, the vessels become less flexible. The vessel is now limited in its ability to expand and deliver an adequate amount of oxygen.

Now there's a gathering of foam cells, lipids, and calcium deposits. This enlarging bump becomes further oxygen deprived and develops a necrotic center made up of dead cells within the *atherosclerotic plaque*. Plaque tends to affect larger arteries, making their walls brittle and weak. If inflammation persists, the plaque becomes unstable, ruptures, and sends its contents out into the blood vessel. Platelets gather around the ruptured plaque, causing a clot (made up of red blood cells and platelets) in the lumen of the blood vessel and obstructing the blood flow. Studies show that this combination of ruptured plaque and blood clot (*thrombus*) accounts for the majority (95 percent) of heart attacks in the world. It's why so many heart attacks happen without any warning and why aspirin, which deactivates platelets and prevents clotting, provides some protection from them.

> **TIPS:** *Heart attack survivors and people with higher risk for heart attack should ask their physicians about taking low-dose aspirin. You should not take aspirin if you are at risk for gastrointestinal bleeding or hemorrhagic stroke, are a heavy alcohol drinker, or are undergoing any surgical or dental procedure. If you have heart attack warning signs, you should call 911 immediately, and the operator may recommend you take aspirin while waiting for emergency medical technicians. Taking daily supplements like vitamin E, ginseng, and Chinese herbs may be beneficial due to their blood-thinning ability.*

Problems Can Begin Early in Life

While atherosclerosis and arteriosclerosis used to be considered unavoidable diseases of aging, both can begin fairly early in life, long before you get your first invitation to AARP. Most life-threatening circulation problems don't arise spontaneously. They are years in the making, stemming from constant assault to our blood vessels that cause circulation issues that are invisible in a routine physical exam or even to some invasive tests. Many of us have

[11]

atherosclerosis or arteriosclerosis with no symptoms; we don't even realize the chronic disease of our blood vessels may be taking a toll on our bodies. Even when asymptomatic, atherosclerosis and arteriosclerosis can cause inadequate blood flow to any part of the body, leading to a shortage of oxygen and nutrients needed for cellular metabolism.

In scientific literature, the two terms *arteriosclerosis* and *atherosclerosis* are used interchangeably and often referred to as *atherosclerosis*. Atherosclerosis without discernible symptoms can still result in cardiovascular disease, but new studies also show links to many seemingly random issues, such as cognitive impairment and early baldness. There's even a link between atherosclerosis and cancer.

A Canadian study shows that a staggering proportion of young, presumably healthy adults who have a normal body weight and body mass index (BMI) already have atherosclerosis[2]. That study revealed a link between visceral fat—abdominal fat hidden deep in the abdomen or chest—and atherosclerosis, even when the young person had a normal body weight and BMI.

A US study done in 1993 of car accident fatalities in patients younger than thirty-five year old showed atherosclerotic heart disease in 78 percent of individuals at autopsy. One in five had more than 50 percent narrowing of their vessels. Of the study group, 9 percent already had narrowed their blood vessels by 75 percent—a drastic reduction in blood flow!

> *TIPS: Blood tests and regular physicals should begin in the teenage years and be continued throughout adult life. Exercising, eating fruits and vegetables, and quitting smoking can never begin too early. There are also noninvasive tests to detect atherosclerosis and blood vessel problems, such as novel 3-D vascular ultrasound, but the best test is the cardiac calcium score. Cardiac Calcium Scoring also known as Heart Scan is a noninvasive CT scan of the heart. This imaging test quantifies the buildup of calcium plaque in the coronary arteries and it will give a risk assessment of heart disease.*

A Surgeon's Perspective

Plastic surgeons like me depend on healthy circulation for good outcomes in every surgery they do—reconstructive or cosmetic—which is why I've been paying *a lot* of attention to blood vessels and how blood flows for many years. Plastic surgeons probably know more about the nitty-gritty of blood circulation than any other surgeons. It isn't a surprise that many of the people who come into my office want to look better or younger. The majority of my surgeries involves lifting tissue from one area on a patient's body and moving it to another site, which also means making sure there's a blood supply ready and working to deliver oxygen to the tissue. As I disconnect some blood vessels, I rely on the remaining ones to carry the load. Or sometimes I'll perform grafts, which require new blood vessels to grow. Regardless, if my patients are going to heal after a facelift, tummy tuck, breast reconstruction, or traumatic injury, they need good, healthy blood flow to the surgical site. So blood vessels and blood flow are constantly on my mind. If you don't think circulation is a *major* part of my profession, check out Professor G. Ian Taylor, founder of the Reconstructive Plastic Surgery Research Unit at the University of Melbourne, Australia. His achievements are considered direct descendants of those of the father of circulation, William Harvey. Dr. Taylor is known for his detailed study of blood supply, for identifying and mapping the vascular anatomy of the body so the appropriate blood vessel lifelines are obvious to us as we transfer tissues from one area in the body to another. His contribution to reconstructive surgery has been compared to the impact GPS has had on navigation. Because of his findings, surgeons can more confidently predict results when they are cutting and disconnecting certain blood vessels. Surgical outcomes are much more reliable because we understand the circulatory system.

TIP: If you have a chronic disease like diabetes, high blood pressure, or obesity or if you are a smoker, know that you are at higher risk for complications from any surgery. Chronic diseases create disturbance in the blood flow throughout the entire body. So if you are thinking of having surgery or any procedure, you may need more extensive preoperative preparation to reduce your risk.

[13]

Athletes

To emphasize again just how indispensable our circulatory system is, let's leave science behind for a moment and look to the world of sports. Professional athletes recognize the power of the circulatory system, and some go too far in trying to manipulate oxygen delivery to cells. One well-documented example is Lance Armstrong. For years, Armstrong was considered superhuman, having survived a diagnosis of metastasized testicular cancer in 1996 and then going on to win the ultimate test of cardiovascular fitness and endurance—the twenty-one-day, 2,200-mile bike race tour de France, not just once or twice, but seven times, every year from 1999 to 2005. A grueling passage through the French mountain chains of the Pyrenees and the Alps, including twenty-one stages that include flat, hilly, mountainous, and high-altitude rides and finishes on the Champs-Élysées in Paris, riders must overcome fatigue, illness, weight loss, breathing issues, and possibly even injuries from crashes. For many, winning isn't the goal; finishing is.

The major difficulty with the Tour de France is that the oxygen demand involved in riding such a long and arduous path exceeds that of any sport, taking a toll on blood oxygen levels, the heart, lungs, and blood vessels. That oxygen-delivery system is one of the most limiting but important aspects of an athlete's performance in the race. Cyclists train for many years before participating in the tour and even winning once is a monumental achievement. So how was Lance Armstrong able to win seven times? After years of speculation, in 2012, a decision by the US Anti-Doping Agency and the International Cycling Union stripped him of all seven titles and ended his professional athletic career, stating that Armstrong had used performance-enhancing drugs. In fact, he was named the ringleader of "the most sophisticated, professionalized, and successful doping program that sport has ever seen."

Basically, he manipulated the oxygen-carrying capacity of his red blood cells, and he wasn't alone in doing so. Sometimes he'd withdraw one to four units of his own blood and refrigerate it for several weeks before a race. After allowing his body to build back the red blood cell count, just prior to a race, he would transfuse his own blood, significantly increasing the number of red blood cells coursing through his body. Transfusing this blood increased oxygen

[14]

delivery to his tissues and improved his performance. It also meant that he had more red blood cells in his body than the other riders.

For some races, he was injected with erythropoietin (EPO), a substance that increases red blood cell mass, also allowing more blood to be transported to the muscles. EPO occurs naturally in the body and is released from the kidneys to stimulate red blood cell production in the bone marrow. It is usually used to treat anemia in kidney dialysis patients.

Blood doping is not legal in professional sports. Between 1998 and 2012, one-third of the top ten finishers at the Tour de France tested positive for or admitted to doping, and many in the sport believe that a lot more were involved but never caught.

One legal way to manipulate blood oxygen levels is to train at high altitudes. Evolutionary biologists have observed that one small geographical area, about one-sixtieth of the continent of Africa, is dominant in long-distance running. Runners from Kenya have clocked seven of the ten fastest times ever for marathons (26.2 miles) and are among the most consistent winners in the world, having won marathons in Boston, New York, London, Berlin, Chicago, and Tokyo. Ethiopia boasts Olympic and world champions Haile Gebreselassie and Kenenisa Bekele. During the last five Olympic games, fifty-three of the ninety medals in distance events have gone to runners from Kenya or Ethiopia.

The thin, oxygen-poor air at high altitudes fascinates runners from around the world, and many are moving to locales with altitudes similar to Kenya and Ethiopia. Why? Sparse oxygen forces our bodies to increase their red blood cells, thus increasing the amount of oxygen delivered to muscles during exercise and improving performance. There's also a chemical change within the red blood cells that makes them more efficient at unloading oxygen to tissues. Some call it "natural" EPO. According to USA Track & Field recommendations, athletes should live between seven thousand and eight thousand feet above sea level to maximize oxygen delivery to tissues during competition.

Perhaps you've heard of Novak Djokovic, the Serbian tennis player who spends time in an egg-shaped machine called a *CVAC pod*. During a twenty-minute session, the body is exposed to dynamic pressure changes and lower oxygen levels (simulating high altitude). It works by forcing adaptations in the body, much like physical training. It sends people into a state of oxygen deficiency, and the body responds by producing EPO. Additionally, a protein complex called hypoxia inducible factor (HIF) is released into the bloodstream, which sparks new vessel growth.

Everyday athletes can take advantage of the circulatory system too. A study by researchers at the University of Pisa published in *Circulation* in 2000 compared sedentary individuals to those who were more active and then to athletic individuals as well, looking at the effects of exercise in different age groups. Both groups of young people—sedentary and athletic—had an average age of twenty-seven. In the older group, the sedentary people averaged sixty-three years of age, and the athletes averaged sixty-six years of age. The study found that the blood vessels of the older athletes functioned just as well as those in both of the younger groups, demonstrating that regular physical activity preserves the health of your blood vessels[3].

But you don't have to be athletic to benefit from your circulatory system. Brisk walking, gardening, cleaning a car, and doing daily physical chores are very effective ways to keep the blood vessels flexible. Don't delegate movement to others! The bottom line is to use your own muscles, reap the benefits every day and get the blood flowing.

TIPS: One of the best breathing technique to properly oxygenate your body:
The 4-7-8 Breathing Exercise: Start by sitting up straight with good posture. Exhale completely through your mouth. Close your mouth with the tongue touching the roof of the mouth, Inhale slowly through your nostrils to a count of four. Hold the air in your lungs for count of seven. Finally exhale through the mouth slowly, making a whoosh sound to a count of eight. Repeat the exercise four to five times. You can practice this breathing exercise several times a day. It will relax you and get rid of stale air often trapped in the lungs. If you decide to be more physical, you can fully oxygenate your muscles and clear carbon dioxide from your body by following a 3:2 inhale-to-exhale ratio. Let's say you are running. Inhale for three steps, then exhale for two. Three counts in, two counts out. You will be delivering more oxygen

*to your cells and slowing your heartbeat. If you are exerting
or lifting, always exhale on exertion. When you exhale while
lifting or pushing, you will be protecting blood vessels from
injury.*

Emergencies

What if there is an interruption or hole in the circulatory
system? I know quite a bit about life-threatening circulatory
problems—the kinds that bring patients rushing into an emergency
room or trauma center. Early in my career, I worked as the chief
surgical resident at a major metropolitan hospital in New York City,
a hospital that was a level-one trauma center. Life-threatening
circulatory problems were always the most urgent issues we treated
or consulted on, whether in the emergency room, surgical unit, the
coronary care unit (CCU), or the medical intensive care unit
(MICU).

It was the beginning of the 1990s, and the crime rate was, and
still remains the highest ever reported in New York City. There were
2,245 murders in New York City in 1990. Victims of muggings,
knifings and gunshots were pouring into trauma centers (nicknamed
"knife and gun clubs" by medical staff) and the crack epidemic was
in full swing. Adding to the high trauma numbers was the fact that
airbags were not yet routinely built into cars.

Many people may not realize that the first sixty minutes after
a bullet blasts through a spleen, a knife is thrust into a belly, or a
steering wheel crushes a sternum are crucial. Those of us in medicine
call it the "golden hour" or "platinum minutes." Our priority in the
trauma center was to stabilize blood pressure and restore normal
circulation for all these patients as quickly as possible, because we
knew that ensuring blood flow to the vital organs was essential to
minimizing permanent damage.

In the trauma center, our first task with injured patients was
to do an ABC assessment—airway, breathing, and *circulation*—
emergency protocol that was established by Mobile Army Surgical
Hospitals (MASH) during the Korean and Vietnam Wars. ABC
assessments saved the lives of a significant number of soldiers and
transformed trauma care in the United States. We knew that if a
patient's circulatory system had been disrupted, that patient was in
real danger of dying.

[17]

Everything we did in the initial trauma assessment was aimed at ensuring that oxygen was getting to the lungs, into the circulatory system, and being delivered to organs, tissues, and cells throughout the body. First, we'd quickly establish that nothing was obstructing the flow of oxygen to the lungs. Second, we'd make sure the patient could breathe on his or her own, and if not, we'd provide assistance. Finally, and most importantly, we'd check the blood flow, or *hemodynamics*, by measuring the patient's pulse, blood pressure, and oxygen saturation to ensure the circulatory system was functioning.

In the world of trauma centers and facilities for military personnel at war, restoring circulation is recognized as the number-one priority in saving a life.

> **TIP:** *If you accidentally cut off a finger, be sure to wrap it in gauze and put it in a bag of ice. The ice will preserve the finger. Then, get to an emergency room as soon as you can with the wrapped finger. If it is reattached quickly, the circulation can be restored to save the finger.*

Chapter 2: How Our Circulation Impacts the Body

Here's an important notion, and one that I hope will affect your decisions regarding nutrition, movement, and exposure to toxins: blood flow is involved in every aspect of your life—the way you look, feel, think, and move. There's nothing that is more important than protecting and promoting healthy blood flow. Nothing.

Let's take a closer look at how circulation affects every part of your body.

Skin

Your skin is your body's barrier against the outside world, your protection, and it provides a first impression about your appearance. You carry around eight pounds of skin; that's twenty-two square feet of skin, which is made of two layers—epidermis, on the outside, and dermis, on the inside.

There's a network of small blood vessels in your skin that contain muscles in their walls. Controlled by the nervous system, these vessels can expand and contract, allowing the skin to regulate your body temperature. When they contract, less blood flows to your skin, which helps keep heat in your body. That's why, when it's cold outside, less blood flows to the surface of your skin and makes you look paler. When the vessels relax or expand, blood flows to the skin, taking heat away from the core and out of your body. When blood is flowing to your skin, it looks flushed, healthy, vibrant, and glowing.

As you grow older, your skin changes, resulting in sagging, crow's feet, and wrinkles. By the time you hit forty, your skin might begin thickening in the *stratum corneum* (the very outside layer of the epidermis). That's the part you see in the mirror, and it's mostly made of dead cells and a little collagen. The older we get, the drier, flakier and denser it gets. At the same time, the *dermis* (deeper layer of skin) becomes thinner as collagen turnover decreases and skin loses its elasticity. Skin becomes more fragile and much more prone to injury and disease. These changes happen whether your skin is sun damaged or not; they just happen with age and the passage of time.

But what if you have poor circulation as well? It can leave skin looking pallid and dull, with pigmentation, dark spots, and

[19]

blotches. Poor circulation means less oxygen, fewer nutrients, and less white blood cell flow to the skin, resulting in slower healing and less collagen production, which translates to more wrinkles.

The good news here is that your skin can look more youthful, and you don't have to slather it with expensive creams. As it turns out, healthy circulation keeps skin younger, and research shows that a focus on exercise and nutrition may even reverse skin aging in people who start exercising late in life.

In one study presented at the American Medical Society for Sports Medicine, researchers at McMasters University assembled twenty-nine male and female volunteers between the ages of twenty and eighty-four. Half of the volunteers were active, exercising for about three hours a week, and the other half led much more sedentary lives and exercised less than half an hour per week. To determine how exercise affects skin quality, each of the participants had a sample taken from their buttocks, an area of the body not regularly exposed to the sun.

Researchers took the skin samples and found that when compared strictly by age, they were pretty much as expected—older volunteers mostly had thicker outer layers of skin and thinner inner layers. But a closer look revealed that, in volunteers over the age of forty, those who had been physically active had thinner, healthier stratum corneum and thicker dermis. The skin composition looked more like that of a twenty- or thirtysomething, even if the participant was over the age of sixty-five!

To further test this, they asked a group of volunteers over sixty-five who were not physically active to start exercising. Before the study, they had "normal" skin for their age. They were placed on a moderately strenuous exercise program, jogging or cycling twice a week for thirty minutes. In just three months' time, when skin samples were examined under a microscope, they looked significantly different; their dermis and epidermis looked like a twenty- to forty-year-old's!

Another study confirmed that exercise improved blood flow to the skin by increasing the production of nitric oxide (resulting in vasodilation). Robust circulation makes skin healthier and look younger. Cancer research even showed exercise reduced skin cancer in animal models (more on this in the cancer section).

TIPS: Antiaging and antioxidant creams are big business. They remove and smooth the skin from the outside. The effects are temporary, and they may make you feel better, but if you really want to get your skin glowing, go for a nice run or a bike ride. This will enhance the blood flow to your skin and cleanse the skin from the inside. You will start to see immediate improvement in your skin color and texture that will last.

For an added boost, eating ginger root can stimulate circulation. It decreases inflammation and brings more oxygen and nutrients to the skin. Ginkgo biloba is another natural supplement that can improve your circulation, and it is available in capsules.

Heart

Ah, the heart. Beating away under our ribcages, slightly to the left of our breastbones and between our lungs. A giant muscle the size of our fist, it pumps blood continually to every inch of our body. It is the fulcrum of our circulatory system, the maestro conducting its orchestra with precision so every cell will be fed with oxygen-rich blood. The heart is central to both the plumbing and electrical aspects of our physiology.

The heart is both fed with blood (through coronary arteries) and feeds the rest of the body by pumping blood. The left and right atria are smaller chambers that pump blood into the ventricles. The left and right ventricles are stronger pumps. First, the right atrium receives oxygen-poor blood from the body and pumps it to the right ventricle through the tricuspid valve. Next, the right ventricle pumps the oxygen-poor blood to the lungs through the pulmonary valve. Third, the left atrium receives oxygen-rich blood from the lungs and pumps it to the left ventricle through the mitral valve. Finally, the more muscular left ventricle pumps the oxygen-rich blood through the aortic valve out to the entire body.

In a normally functioning heart, all four chambers synchronize contractions to keep oxygen-rich blood circulating throughout the body. It's a big job and requires the heart to
• regulate the timing of the heartbeat through a sophisticated electrical system,

- contract and relax so it can fill with blood and then pump it into the body, and
- keep blood flowing efficiently through the heart valves.

If any of those functions go wrong, the outcome can be disastrous. One or more of the valves may start leaking, allowing blood to flow backward; this is called *regurgitation*. Valves can also become stiffer over time (*stenosis*) and this can restrict blood flow through the heart. Sometimes there is trouble with the electrical impulses that dictate heart contraction. If the heart does not receive impulses in a regular manner, the contractions can be ineffective in coordinating the blood flow. The most common problem in the heart, however, is when the coronary arteries get blocked, causing blood flow to the heart muscles to slow or stop.

Even if you've never had a heart attack, you may have experienced what it feels like when there's a momentary lapse in oxygen delivery to your heart. Temporary chest pain is referred to as *angina*. It occurs during stress or exercise as a result of the heart not getting enough oxygen. Angina happens when there is an underlying heart problem and one or more coronary arteries are partially blocked or narrowed. The heart is sending out a signal that you should stop what you are doing immediately.

Instant relief can come from nitroglycerin, a potent vasodilator, being given under the tongue. The drug is quickly converted to nitric oxide, which relaxes large blood vessels, so the heart doesn't have to pump as hard. Ultimately, nitroglycerin reduces the heart's workload.

What happens during a heart attack, also called a *myocardial infarction* (MI)? When there is a blockage of a coronary artery carrying blood to the heart, damage to the heart muscle can occur. A partial blockage can progress to a complete blockage without warning. Plaque can break off, causing a clot to form, stopping oxygen-rich blood to that part of the heart. Once this happens, there is irreversible damage to that area of the heart.

The heart is the focal point of our circulatory system, but it is also the most vulnerable part. Even a brief interruption in blood flow to the heart can have catastrophic consequences, so always be mindful and protect your heart!

TIP: The most common symptom of a heart attack is intense pressure or squeezing on the chest, or chest pain that lasts more than few minutes or goes away and then comes back. But it can also manifest as pain radiating to the arms, back, neck, jaw, or even to the stomach. In women, shortness of breath may be the first sign. Some may experience cold sweat, nausea, or lightheadedness. Don't ignore these symptoms!

Liver

Liver doesn't grab headlines, but behind the scenes, it performs many duties that are critical to our survival. The largest solid organ in the body, it wears many different hats. The ultimate multitasker, it's estimated to have over five hundred separate functions. The liver is our very own chemical processing plant—it is involved in metabolism and energy production, regulation of blood sugar level, lipid metabolism (including making cholesterol), protein and hormone synthesis, bile production; storage of vitamin A, D, E, K, B, iron, and copper; blood clotting, and detoxification of toxins. *The liver's reach is vast and irreplaceable.*

The liver weighs roughly three pounds and is about the size of a football; it is located in the right upper quadrant of the abdomen, protected by the rib cage. It has dual blood supply: the hepatic artery bringing oxygen-rich blood from the heart and the portal vein delivering nutrients from the entire GI tract. It acts as a secondary defense after the pathogens and toxins pass through the GI barrier by the neutralizing effect of Kupffer cells (these are immune cells that eliminate residual foreign invaders). However, essential functions of the organ are carried out by the hepatocytes, the most abundant liver cells. The liver is the only visceral organ in our bodies capable of regeneration (it can grow to full size from as little as 25 percent of the original mass in just 8 to 15 days). A recent study found that the size of the liver even oscillates throughout the day depending on its activity, swelling and shrinking.

All food you eat must go through the liver before it is converted into energy. The liver maintains metabolic homeostasis (equilibrium) by keeping sugar level constant in our bloodstream. It is able to store sugar as glycogen (about 400 calories worth) and regulates blood sugar by releasing glycogen when the sugar level drops. It also converts excess sugar into fat after the glycogen tank is full and can breakdown stored fat and convert it to fuel in times of starvation. *The liver implements both fat storage and fat burning.*

All problems in the liver arise from those cells not getting enough oxygen. This should sound familiar. The most common cause in developed countries is due to fat deposits called *non-alcoholic fatty liver disease;* in the United States, 30 to 40 percent of adults are already living with this disease. With weight gain, the excess fat goes everywhere in the body, including the organs. As the liver becomes embedded with fat, the blood flow slows.

Another cause of fatty liver is excess alcohol consumption. Other liver disease can come from viral infection (hepatitis), injury from toxins, or autoimmune attack. No matter the origin of the liver injury, they all run through the common channel of chronic inflammation leading to compromised delivery of oxygen and nutrients. As more and more liver cells become damaged, they're replaced with scar tissues; this condition is called *liver fibrosis.* When liver cells are choked off from oxygen supply, they begin to die and result in *cirrhosis.* Once this occurs the liver cells sustain irreversible damage. Studies show that in all liver disease, there is marked reduction in the blood flow to the liver cells. Furthermore, when liver cells are oxygen deprived, cancer risk goes way up. If the liver fails, the only way to restore liver function is through a transplant.

TIPS: When it comes to the health of your body, don't let the liver take the back seat. Liver disease can affect people of all shapes and sizes. Be proactive and you can reverse the damage. You can check your liver enzymes, called LFTs, in your blood test at least once a year. If you're overweight or if you have elevated blood sugar, you may already have liver damage. Losing weight can reduce fatty liver disease and decrease liver inflammation.

Cut down your alcohol consumption and inflammation will begin to subside. Alcoholic fatty liver may resolve within six weeks if you stop drinking.

If you have viral hepatitis (B or C), taking antiviral meds will keep the virus from injuring your liver. You can monitor it by following your viral count.

Fibroscan can be done to determine the stage/severity of liver disease. It is a noninvasive ultrasound to assess the extent of scarring and fat deposits in the liver. Stop ingesting toxins and drugs. Common drugs that can harm your liver include Tylenol (acetaminophen), ibuprofen, aspirin, steroids, and statins. Avoid direct contact with cleaning and aerosol products. Supplements and herbs are not always beneficial; some may be toxic to your liver.

Mental Health

The adult brain weighs approximately three pounds, which is about 2 percent of our entire body weight. Yet even on a lazy day, the brain consumes 20 percent of all the energy being used by your body. If your total daily energy expenditure is 2000 calories, then your brain alone is burning 400 calories just doing very basic tasks. The brain also contains over 100,000 miles of a vast network of blood vessels. It is highly dependent on oxygen—brain cells start dying after only five minutes without it!

Oxygen and nutrients are carried to the brain by the many blood vessels on the surface and deep within the brain. Blood vessels (and nerves) enter the brain through holes in the skull called *foramina.*

The brain needs 20 percent of the body's blood supply to keep the body functioning and oversee motor control, visual and auditory processing, sensation, learning, memory, and emotions. Since the brain is the command center of the body, it gets top priority when it comes to blood allocation.

Two pairs of arteries serve as the delivery service—the internal carotid arteries and the vertebral arteries. They join at the base of the brain and form a ring of arteries called the *circle of Willis.* The circle of Willis is the brain's ingenious safety mechanism—if one of the arteries gets blocked, the "circle" will ensure that blood still flows to the brain. Any interruption or delay in the blood flow to your brain significantly impacts your mental health, especially issues of depression and cognitive function.

As we age, our brains shrink, and that creates a space between the brain surface and the skull. Cavities that hold cerebrospinal fluid enlarge, nerve tracts shrivel, and brain circuitry is reduced. These natural processes lead to decline in cognitive function and an incline in depression.

Beyond brain shrinkage, diminished blood flow from inflexible, small vessels that are more easily clogged can cause ministrokes of which we may not even be aware. If brain cells are injured or infected, healthy neurons are bombarded by inflammatory chemicals, like cytokines. *Cytokines* are an immune system response that can further damage the brain and affect behavioral and cognitive abilities.

You shouldn't be surprised by what slows blood flow or causes inflammation in the brain: anything that affects our health, like excess body fat, smoking, poor diet, and chronic disease. Research has shown that people who suffer various chronic diseases, such as heart, liver, and lung disease, have much higher rates of depression and cognitive function decline. People are also more prone to depression following a stroke.

In patients with depression, studies show that there is decreased blood flow to the brain and a drop in serotonin levels. When depression lifts, blood flow is restored and serotonin levels rise. Antidepressants and psychotherapy both help stabilize impaired blood flow to the brain, according to brain imaging research.

What this also comes down to is that circulation is very important to your mental health. Even a small reduction of blood flow can lower comprehension abilities and trigger headaches, dizziness, and forgetfulness. As blood flow slows more dramatically, studies show people often suffer paranoia, short-term memory loss, and confusion.

Studies dating back to 1981 have shown that regular exercise can boost the moods of people with mild or moderate depression and may even help treat severe depression. Some studies show that exercise is a viable substitute for people who wish to avoid taking antidepressants. While it may take longer to see mood changes and it may be difficult to maintain the level of physical activity, findings have shown that consistent exercise has longer-lasting effects than antidepressants[4].

So how much exercise does it take to reap the mental benefits? A study published in 2005 found that walking fast for about thirty-five minutes a day five times a week or sixty minutes a day three times a week could have a significant effect on mild to moderate depression. But walking fifteen minutes a day, five times a week or doing stretching exercises did not ease depression.

While speeding up blood flow, exercise also promotes the action of endorphins (chemicals that circulate through the body and can enhance natural immunity and reduce pain perception). Exercise also stimulates the release of neurotransmitters called *serotonin* and *norepinephrine*, which may directly improve mood. The physical benefits of exercise—lowered blood pressure, protection against heart disease and cancer, and raised self-esteem—can all benefit mental health.

How you fuel your brain matters as well. Foods can affect how the blood flows into your brain. Diets high in refined sugar can worsen the body's regulation of insulin and promote inflammation and oxidative stress (free radicals), damaging blood vessels all over the body, including in the brain. Many studies show a direct relationship between refined sugars and impaired brain function and depression. Unfortunately, it has taken quite a long time for the medical community to make this connection.

TIPS: The brain is made of 60 percent fat, and it depends on dietary fats to replenish its supply. Eating good amounts of essential fatty acids—fats that cannot be synthesized by our body, like omega-3—will optimize our mental health. Healthy fats include fatty fish like salmon, nuts, avocados, and seeds. Daylight also has been proven to fight off depression. Enjoy sunlight when you can but consider changing your light bulbs to natural daylight bulbs.

Vision

The human eye has been called the most complex organ in the body, as well as your window to the world. So what can we do to protect our eyesight? The truth is, despite your best efforts, your vision will deteriorate as you age. While most of these changes can be corrected either with surgery or prescriptive lenses, two eye diseases that affect tens of millions of Americans are the most common causes of blindness in the elderly and the adult. The first, affecting the elderly population is called *age-related macular degeneration* (AMD) and refers to the breakdown of the macula—a densely concentrated collection of special light-sensing cells in the

[27]

central portion of the retina. The macula provides our eyes with sharp, forward vision.

The job of the retina is to receive visual signals, do a quick analysis of them, transmit the information to the brain, and produce an image. A rich network of blood vessels carries oxygen and vital nutrients that are required for healthy vision, and any change in these vessels can be a contributing factor in retinal injury. The retina has no pain receptors; therefore, most diseases that affect the retina do not cause pain.

The second disease, rapidly rising among adults, is called *diabetic retinopathy* (DR) and occurs from high blood sugar wreaking havoc on the blood vessels nourishing the retina. The architecture of the blood vessels is abnormal and dysfunctional in the retinas of both AMD and DR, thereby profoundly reducing the oxygen level. Anything that interrupts, slows, or interferes with flow of blood can adversely impact the retina. Not surprisingly this is same list that causes atherosclerosis: smoking, obesity, diabetes, unhealthy diet, and a loss of antioxidants.

> *TIP: Get regular eye exams. Prescription changes are normal, but losing vision is not. Researchers have known for decades that people who consume food rich in vitamin C, vitamin E, and zinc have much lower risk of vision loss. Vitamin C–rich foods are fruits and cruciferous vegetables like broccoli, while foods rich in vitamin E are leafy greens, nuts, seeds, avocados, shellfish, and fish. Foods with high levels of zinc are seafood, wheat germs, spinach, nuts, and beans. Food containing these ingredients helps promote healthy blood vessels and protects the retina against free radical damage.*

Hair

Since Samson and Delilah, hair has represented youth and vitality in our culture. And in our quest for beauty, we in the United States spend upwards of $15 billion on hair care products alone! And that figure doesn't include the money spent in hair salons and products sold in those salons. In other cultures around the world, hair represents social status, sensuality, a connection to the spirit and so much more. It's clear that hair is more than just filament.

There are four phases of hair growth: anagen, catagen, telogen, and exogen. Hair cycles through periods of growth and rest. Although it spends the majority of the time in the growth phase (anagen), your hair spends more time in the resting phase (telogen) as you get older, contributing to thinning of the hair. It's true that genetic components can lead to baldness in men, and stress and medication can cause your hair to fall out. But as new hair grows, it requires good amounts of nutrients and a toxin-free environment. So keeping yourself healthy and having optimal circulation can give you the best hair possible.

Our hair follicles rely on an abundant supply of blood flow, constantly bringing with them oxygen and nutrients. A study from Denmark found that the scalp of men with early male pattern baldness had markedly decreased blood flow compared to the normal control subjects[5]. Subsequent studies found significantly lower levels of oxygen in the balding areas of those with male pattern baldness.

What about Rogaine (minoxidil) for hair growth in men? While the exact way it works is not known for sure, it is a vasodilator, meaning when applied topically on the scalp, it delivers more blood (and shortens the resting phase). Increased blood flow helps improve hair follicle function and stimulates cell growth. Pretty simple stuff, right?

Researchers at Massachusetts General Hospital have been able to enhance hair growth on mice. By using a protein called vascular endothelial growth factor (VEGF), they were able to stimulate blood vessels to grow—augmenting delivery of oxygen and nutrients to the skin. The mice were able to grow their hair faster and thicker. Although the number of hair follicles was not affected, there was a dramatic 70 percent increase in volume, resulting in fuller hair.

While blood flow to the scalp may not impact the quantity of hair growth, it certainly affects the quality. The thin, wispy, see-through hair seen in both men and women in their late fifties and beyond can be partly attributed to circulation issues.

TIPS: Sixty-day scalp massage challenge: Massage your scalp once a day for five to ten minutes for thirty days, then twice a day (morning and night) for an additional thirty days. For many years barbers have known the benefits of scalp massages. Studies have shown that massaging your scalp will stimulate the blood flow to the scalp, producing thicker hair. Continue to massage your scalp for five minutes twice a day for maintenance. In addition, micro-needling (or derma roller)—a procedure that is used to rejuvenate the skin by creating multiple small punctures on the scalp—may also promote blood flow and stimulate collagen synthesis. Recently published reports have shown that micro needling— when combined with Rogaine—was superior to treatment with Rogaine alone for hair growth.

Sexual Function

Blood goes everywhere in your body, right? But what about those intimate times when not enough gets to where you need it most? When the lights are low and the mood is right, erectile dysfunction can strike, meaning that a man can't have sex because he cannot get or keep an erection. It affects 30 percent of men between the ages of forty and seventy—up to thirty million men in the United States alone. And while it can be caused by depression, low testosterone, a nerve problem, or even some medications, it is atherosclerosis, inability of blood to flow that is responsible in the majority of cases. That's right. You can now also apply Poiseuille's law to your sex life. Small changes in the size of the arteries in the penis—due to plaque buildup, blockage, or the inability to expand— can lead to erectile dysfunction.

As we covered earlier, when your arteries harden and cannot dilate due to injury to the endothelial cells (lining the blood vessels) by toxins and inflammation, blood flow slows. Usually, the penis is the first organ to notice the slow flow, which is why erectile dysfunction can actually be a warning sign that something more life-threatening could happen in the next five years—like a heart attack or a stroke.

Sexual dysfunction was first researched and studied in the 1950s by the team of William Masters and Virginia Johnson at Washington University in St. Louis. Pioneers in their field, with extensive research dedicated to the nature of sexual response in humans, their research and publications (*Human Sexual Response,*

1966 and *Human Sexual Inadequacy*, 1970) opened up a public discussion on sexuality. In 1970, the pair appeared on the cover of the May 25 *TIME Magazine* with a headline that announced a new sex education for adults. Physicians and therapists started studying their therapeutic approach to sexual dysfunction, and almost overnight, couple's therapy was all the rage. They introduced America to female sexual prowess, argued that clitoral stimulation was involved in all the female orgasms, and debunked what Freud had written on this topic. They developed couple's therapy that involved sensate touching exercises and communication to combat problems like erectile dysfunction. These innovations provided the country with new understandings of sex, new sexual expectations, and a new focus on female sexuality. Ironically, they also inspired the development of a little blue pill (Viagra) that would deal the deathblow to those very ideas.

The pharmaceutical industry was aware of the wide interest in the pair's research and claims about sexual dysfunction. Pfizer Pharmaceuticals realized a huge financial opportunity upon the discovery that a medication they were testing as a treatment for angina also caused erections. The FDA approved the use of sildenafil citrate (marketed as Viagra) as the first oral pill to treat impotence on March 27, 1998. Here's how it works:

Sildenafil regulates blood flow to the penis. It does not cause sexual arousal, however, if a man is sexually aroused, the nervous system in the tissue of his penis releases nitric oxide, which stimulates an enzyme that produces something called a *messenger cyclic guanosine monophosphate* (cGMP). The cGMP relaxes the smooth muscle in the arteries of the penis—or vasodilation—so the arteries open wider and blood can flood into the penis and the erectile tissues. Viagra and other drugs, like Cialis, and Levitra, prevent a naturally existing enzyme called PDE5 from breaking down cGMP, so the vasodilation process is enhanced; the arteries in the penis dilate, allowing blood to flow there more easily. Since blood flow problems to the genitalia occur with aging in both sexes, Viagra has also been successful in treating women with sexual dysfunction. By improving the blood flow to the genital area, it increases the sensation of warmth, tingling, and fullness, leading to a better orgasm.

[31]

TIPS: Anything that is bad for your heart is also bad for sexual function. Smoking, high-sugar and processed food diets, excess weight—it's all about the blood flow. Having a healthy lifestyle will lead to optimal sexual function. Anything that causes blood vessel disease will lead to sexual dysfunction. Refrain from smoking, incorporate some exercise into your life, eat well, and you will see a substantial improvement in your sex life.

Strong Muscles

We need good blood flow to keep our muscles nourished with oxygen and nutrients, and if there is a disruption, then all the muscles in our body will suffer. Just as the heart is mostly muscle, a brief interruption in the blood flow may lead to a heart attack (a portion of heart muscle dies).

The muscles that move our arms and legs are the biggest muscles in the body and building them up is like adding horsepower to a car. They will burn more fuel (sugar), therefore lowering our blood sugar. Healthy muscles rev up our metabolism. This doesn't necessarily require bodybuilding or body sculpting. Maintaining healthy muscles by walking briskly, doing daily chores, playing sports, doing yoga, or lifting some light weights can create healthy muscle. If we don't use our muscles, they will atrophy, and eventually the ability to be fully physically active will be gone.

As we age, our energy expenditure lowers because we naturally lose lean muscle mass and end up burning fewer calories. *Sarcopenia*, the natural loss of muscle, begins in our thirties and continues throughout our later years; we lose about one pound of muscle every year. As a result, the body becomes less effective at burning sugar. Our metabolic rate reduces by about 2 percent or more per decade after age twenty-five. At fifty, our metabolism is approximately 5 to 10 percent slower than it was when we were twenty-five. To combat this, we must build more muscle, which will, in turn, amp up our metabolism.

Another benefit of healthy muscles and good blood flow is strong bones. Keeping muscles strong is a great way to prevent osteoporosis and fractures, and to maintain our height as we age. Bones require constant force to retain their density and strength. Contracting muscles provide the resistance that preserves the integrity of the bone. People who are bedridden suffer profound bone loss because they don't exercise the muscles that build skeletal strength. It is interesting to note that astronauts living in a zero-gravity environment suffer similar bone loss due to the lack of force exerted on their bones. Studies have also shown that compromised blood flow to the lower extremities was associated with loss of bone mineral density and osteoporosis.

Brisk blood flow is essential to all the muscles in our bodies, but nowhere is it more important than in our legs. The legs are our workhorses; they need lots and lots of oxygen. If our leg muscles don't receive enough blood, then we may feel pain or cramping while walking called *claudication*. When people are experiencing claudication, they may believe it is a sign of aging, but it's not. It's actually a circulation problem, involving atherosclerosis in the leg. Left untreated, it can lead to ulcers, infections, or loss of limbs. Claudication is a late sign that the blood vessels in our leg are obstructed or can't dilate.

> *TIPS:* *You can check for a pulse in your legs and feet. The best place to feel for a pulse in the leg is just behind the inner anklebone, at your posterior tibial artery. If the pulse is absent, it means you have problem with circulation in your legs. You must see a doctor immediately.*
>
> *You may also have a circulation problem if you experience changes in the color of skin to your feet, if you feel coolness, if you experience pain, if you have loss of hair, or if cuts don't seem to heal properly. If you experience any of these, have it checked out quickly. Early intervention—such as a good exercise program and lifestyle adjustment—can prevent the progression of atherosclerosis and get the blood to your legs and feet flowing.*

Chapter 3: Factors That Influence Our Circulation

Scientists have been trying to figure out what factors negatively impact the circulatory system for decades. We hear a lot about cholesterol being guilty of clogging up the blood vessels and causing heart attacks, but that idea is in question now. Below are the major culprits that work to undermine your circulatory system.

Inflammation

Inflammation is the buzzword of the day, but what does it really mean?

If we look as far back as five hundred million years into our past, we'll see that our primitive ancestors were equipped with an elaborate defense mechanism that protected them from injury, bacteria, viruses, allergens, and toxins—what we call *inflammation*. You know it as pain, swelling, redness, heat, and loss of mobility. It's not fun, but it's essential to healing. Think of your *-itis* ailments—arthritis, gastritis, appendicitis, laryngitis, hepatitis, bursitis, gingivitis, sinusitis… The list goes on and on.

These are all forms of inflammation: *-itis* means inflammation. Usually, acute inflammation lasts only 24–48 hours as the white blood cells, called *neutrophils*, kick in and do their job fighting off infection. The body increases blood flow to the injured area—that's why it gets red and hot—and the blood vessels become more permeable, so the immune system can enter the tissue, which is why you get the swelling.

A compound called *bradykinin* helps the blood vessel dilate and increase blood flow to an injured area. It also makes the vessels more porous by binding to pain receptors. Pain often tells us we've got an injury or an infection. Destroying any invading pathogens and ridding the area of debris, our immune system does its job and then leaves the scene—this is acute inflammation, which is short-lived.

Inflammation is absolutely vital to our survival. Without it, our bodies would be infested with numerous invaders that would ultimately destroy us. By recognizing what is not part of our own bodies, the process of inflammation eliminates what is foreign. It then prepares us for repair and healing.

That's how inflammation is *supposed* to work. But sometimes things go awry, and it happens in places you can't see or feel, or even in places where there's no injury or infection—that's chronic inflammation. It's what happens when our bodies continues to trigger the release of inflammatory messengers that activate our immune systems and never shut off.

The body receives a signal that there's a problem, and it sends out its regular cleaning crew of proteins. But there is no major injury or infection to clean up. Instead there is a persistent irritation from insults or toxins. Confused, the body keeps sending out crews of the proteins to deal with the perceived threat. And they start backing up, creating a traffic jam of sorts in the blood vessels, causing buildup, havoc, and, ultimately, inflammation that doesn't clear out and go away but just hangs around. The existence of a certain protein (C-reactive protein) on the cleaning crew is one of the most notable biomarkers of chronic inflammation and it is also a better indicator of cardiovascular disease than elevated low-density lipoprotein, LDL (LDL which is also known as "bad cholesterol" and has been used as a traditional marker for heart disease for many years).

What initiates this built-in immune response that leads to chronic inflammation? Occasionally, genetics, but more frequently, it's things you have control over, like weight and excess body fat, highly processed food, high blood sugar and insulin levels, smoking, radiation, stress, and environmental toxins.

For instance, sugary diets, refined flours, and trans fats—which can contribute to obesity—also contribute to chronic inflammation. Heck, just eating too much and gaining belly fat can start the process. So can stress, chronic infection from virus, bacteria, yeast or parasites, a lack of exercise, processed food, and environmental allergies. Pesticides, mercury, and molds can also lead to chronic inflammation. Anything that sets off our immune response but never heals enough for it to shut down can lead to chronic inflammation.

What's so destructive about chronic inflammation is that it reduces blood flow to each individual cell. How does it do that? During inflammation, the smallest of the blood vessels, the capillaries, can become injured and even collapse. So even if the oxygen-rich blood makes it all the way into an organ, it may not be able to make the final journey to the cells. When cells don't get enough oxygen, they may shrink, they may multiply, they may

[35]

change, or they may die. Even mild chronic inflammation can reduce the oxygen delivery to cells profoundly. And that can lead to atherosclerosis, heart disease, diabetes, stroke, Alzheimer's, and even cancer.

TIPS: Foods that inflame include refined carbohydrates such as white bread, pastries, soda, sugar-sweetened beverages, also french fries, other fried foods and processed meats (hot dogs and sausages), and processed and packaged foods with hard-to-pronounce ingredients (that is, chemicals). Foods that fight inflammation include olive oil; green, leafy vegetables such as spinach, kale, and collards; nuts like almonds and walnuts; fatty fish like salmon, mackerel, and sardines; and fruits such as strawberries, blueberries, cherries, and oranges.

Brushing your teeth three times a day along with daily flossing is mandatory in reducing gingivitis. Following good oral hygiene routine will lower your overall inflammatory level.

Several tests done together can give your doctor better insight into the degree of inflammation inside your body. Ask for your level of C-reactive protein (and also high-sensitivity C-reactive protein), which is a marker for inflammation but not specific to where the inflammation is occurring. Also test for myeloperoxidase, an enzyme that is more specific to heart disease. Lipid profile (LDL, HDL, triglyceride) is another important piece of the puzzle in assessing your overall inflammation.

Cholesterol

Researchers have finally come to the conclusion that cholesterol is not the bad guy—it does not cause circulation problems, heart attacks, strokes, and more. So what is it? First of all, cholesterol is the best-known and most-abundant steroid found in the body, is in every single cell, and is essential to keeping us alive. Although it is waxy and fatlike, contrary to popular belief, cholesterol is produced by our body—it's not some evil poison only found in certain foods. It's in brain tissue, nerve tissue, and the bloodstream. It helps create the outer coating of cells, and it is the major compound found in bile acids that allow us to digest fat. Our memories are dependent on it. Cholesterol is absolutely necessary to performing basic bodily functions. Our body makes vitamin D, cortisol, and hormones like estrogen and testosterone directly from cholesterol.

We need cholesterol to live!

Our liver is churning out a lot of cholesterol all day long—about 1000+ milligrams of it every day. Nearly 80 percent of the cholesterol in our bodies comes from our livers; the other 20 percent from food we eat. The cholesterol we get from food isn't absorbed by our bodies so well and is quickly excreted. That means that the amount of cholesterol we eat doesn't have that much to do with the cholesterol levels in our bloodstreams, because our livers are actually regulating cholesterol levels by creating more or less of it based on how much of it is needed by our body.

And yet, we hear a lot about "good" cholesterol and "bad" cholesterol. It's so confusing, right? Here's the truth. Both HDL and LDL cholesterols aren't really cholesterol at all. They are *transporters* that carry fats that include cholesterol, triglyceride, phospholipid and other fats from the bloodstream to the liver and from the liver to the cells. They are not cholesterol! They are fat transporters. The so-called "good" cholesterol or high-density lipoprotein (HDL) taxis the cholesterol and other fats from the bloodstream and delivers it to the liver. The liver recycles and disposes excess cholesterol. Most doctors dub this "good" cholesterol and say the more of it, the better.

Then there's the more notorious, so-called "bad" cholesterol or low-density lipoprotein (LDL) whose job it is to deliver fats from the liver to our cells. LDL lands on the dock called *LDL receptor* at the surface of the cell to deliver cholesterol and other fats. This is exactly what LDL was made to do. But these LDL transporters get a bad rap, and the common perception is that we should have low levels of LDL in our blood—but LDL is actually doing an important job. *We can't live without it!*

New studies show that cholesterol in our bodies may calm inflammation, prevent blood clots, support our immune systems, and prevent diseases that cause mutations in our cells. In our quest to improve blood flow and circulation, we should take note of the fact that cholesterol helps stop inflammation, because we know that

[37]

inflammation is how atherosclerosis (plaque) starts. So how did cholesterol get its bad rap?

As researchers began looking at atherosclerosis, the fact that LDL was frequently spotted at the site of plaque deposits in the blood vessels is what started the bad reputation it got. But now researchers think it was actually on the scene to quell the inflammation. *It wasn't the cause of it.*

For instance, when our bodies experience an infection, inflammation, poor thyroid function, or insulin resistance they can trigger our liver to produce more LDL. LDL delivers cholesterol, triglyceride, phospholipid and other fats to the injured site. The elevated LDL is then used to aid our bodies in the healing process. Most LDL is large and buoyant and *we need it.*

Sometimes LDL production can take a detour when our body encounters a problem, especially when it has difficulty processing sugar (i.e. an elevation in blood sugar level). Our liver begins to make a different kind of LDL called *small, dense LDL.* These smaller, denser LDL carry *less* cholesterol than *large, buoyant LDL.* But because they are oddly shaped, they have a much harder time landing on the docks that were designed to receive them. Instead, they float past the docks, linger around, and often, their small size allows them to slip through the blood vessel walls (*endothelium*), become easily oxidized by free radicals and accelerates a plaque formation.

The takeaway: small, dense LDL is born from problems such as elevated blood sugar. These dangerous LDL actually carry less cholesterol, while they lead to the worsening of plaque in the blood vessels.

You should look at your LDL level as an indicator, rather than a toxic substance.

The truth is that countries in which people have higher-than-average cholesterol also have fewer incidence of heart disease. Cholesterol is not a poison. It's an absolutely essential substance in our bodies. And it's very difficult to lower blood cholesterol by lowering cholesterol in our diet. In 2015, the US Department of Agriculture dropped fatty foods containing cholesterol from its list of "nutrients of concern." That same year, the US Dietary Guidelines Advisory Committee dropped their cautionary advice about dietary cholesterol.

[38]

Popular statin drugs which are given to people with "high" cholesterol levels lower cholesterol, but the real benefit may come from lowering inflammation frequently caused by elevated blood sugar. And studies show that people with the lowest cholesterol as they age are at the highest risk for dementia, brain degeneration, heart disease, and cancer—and more recent findings suggest increase in mortality among elderly population from statin therapy. In 2011, the FDA issued warnings against statin drugs that include the risk of liver injury, memory loss, diabetes, muscle damage, and low testosterone level. A Finnish study from 2015 revealed 46 percent increased chance of developing type 2 diabetes with statin use. Still the idea that cholesterol is bad and statin drugs are good helped earn pharmaceutical companies $16.9 billion in 2012 in the United State alone. While highly controversial, some experts believe statin should be used sparingly as others continue to advocate for wider use.

And to further confuse popular belief, a diet rich in cholesterol does not even necessarily mean you'll end up with elevated cholesterol in your blood. Many researchers now point to consumption of sugar as a major contributor driving atherosclerosis and cardiovascular disease. Cholesterol, on the other hand, is a misunderstood scapegoat that has been vilified for too long.

TIPS: All adults age twenty or older should have their cholesterol, and other traditional risk factors checked every year. You should look at the lipid profile along with other blood tests as a marker. Your test report will show cholesterol levels in milligrams per deciliter of blood (mg/dl). A complete lipid profile will show the following:
Total blood (or serum) cholesterol—Your total cholesterol level is calculated using the following equation:

HDL + LDL + 20% of your triglyceride level

With HDL, higher levels are better. Low HDL can mean higher level of small, dense LDL. This can put you at higher risk for heart disease.
A lower LDL level is considered good for your heart health. If you have high LDL but you also have high HDL, then you don't need to worry; it is the ratio of LDL to HDL that is more important. An elevated LDL number by itself does not

[39]

need to be treated in most people, but you need to investigate and treat the cause.

Triglyceride is the most common type of fat in the body. Normal triglyceride levels vary by age and sex but should be below 150. If you have high levels of triglyceride, it will lead to increased small, dense LDL and put you at higher risk for heart disease and stroke.

LDL subfraction test (particle number): This test will measure the number, size, and density of LDL particles. The actual particle number and the size of LDL will give a much better cardiac-risk assessment than cholesterol level alone— A higher LDL particle number and elevated small, dense LDL results in higher risk while larger particle size reduces risk.

Improving your lipid profile: Statin lowers LDL and overall cholesterol levels. It lowers small, dense LDL, but unfortunately it also lowers more of the large, buoyant LDL (which is the good LDL's). Statin raises the ratio of small, dense LDL and can actually increase the concentration, which leads to higher risk of heart disease. Be aware of these contradicting consequences when considering taking statins. There is a reason for elevation in your cholesterol level—our bodies need cholesterol to fight off infection or inflammation. There is a small group of the population with familial hypercholesterolemia who can benefit from statin therapy; they have very high LDL level due to LDL receptor defect— their bloodstream contains markedly elevated LDL, but their cells receive much less cholesterol.

There are safer ways to improve your cholesterol profile. For instance, lowering consumption of refined carbs and processed foods and losing weight are more effective. Niacin supplement can also improve your cholesterol profile; lower small, dense LDL and lower triglyceride levels. Fish oil containing omega-3 fat also lowers triglyceride level, protecting against the formation of small, dense LDL. Consuming one avocado daily can reduce LDL and particle number. Increasing physical activity will raise HDL levels, lead to larger LDL particle size, and will benefit cardiovascular health.

Sugar

Sugar has been linked to heart disease for well over fifty years. In fact, in 1964, an organization now known as the *Sugar Association* met secretly to organize a campaign to combat the public relations problems created by studies that had begun to emerge linking sugar to heart disease. By 1965, the group had formulated a plan to fund Harvard researchers to write a "review" of the scientific literature. For the equivalent of $48,900 today, the Sugar Association was allowed to provide the studies to be analyzed and had the right to review the Harvard researchers' findings. The end product of that deal was an article published in the *New England Journal of Medicine* that linked fat and cholesterol to heart disease and stated that reducing fat intake was undoubtedly the best way to combat cardiovascular disease.

Fat became the villain. Sugar, sweet and sassy, became a viable substitute, as people tried to eat less fat at breakfast, lunch, and dinner.

The outcome of that article and the resulting dietary changes across America is that chronic conditions like obesity, heart disease, and diabetes have continued to climb. That's because elevated sugar in your bloodstream causes free radical formation and also alters a vital enzyme called nitric oxide synthase, which is needed so blood vessels can expand and deliver more oxygen-rich blood. Sugar sticks to everything in the blood and disrupts its function. It is one of the most common causes of chronic inflammation in our bodies. In addition, high doses of sugar in the blood trigger the liver to go into overdrive, making more triglycerides and storing them as abdominal fat.

While sugar is essential, it is important that blood sugar levels do not spike dramatically after a meal. Some simple sugars are absorbed quickly from the intestine and immediately enter the bloodstream, leading to a sugar spike. Sudden sugar spikes can cause you to become sleepy until your levels return to normal. Any calorie-dense meal that spikes your blood sugar can disturb your body's ability to metabolize those calories, trigger the release of free radicals, cause inflammation, and damage blood vessels. There's a direct link between sugar spikes and heart disease and even neuropathy (damage that occurs to nerves).

[41]

Big swings in your blood sugar after eating—up over 140 mg/dl—can make you feel lousy and increase your risk for a number of serious circulation problems. These sugar spikes are extremely treacherous. In fact, researchers from the Mayo Clinic to Johns Hopkins have shown that high blood sugar spikes within a few hours after eating are more relevant to predicting future diabetes and cardiovascular issues than blood sugar tests done during an eight-hour fast.

Glycemic index
Glycemic index (GI) ranks carbohydrates on a scale of 0 to 100, according to how they raise your blood sugar levels after you eat them. The higher the GI score, the more quickly your blood sugar is elevated after eating. The lower scores are for foods that digest and absorb slowly, and lead to gradual rises in blood sugar and insulin levels. Health advantages for eating lower GI foods include appetite control, reduced insulin levels, and reduced insulin resistance. While the GI index is not an absolute value of what foods are the healthiest, it does give a guideline for how food can elevate blood sugar level. Bottom line, you want to prevent wild swings in blood sugar. Foods containing higher amounts of simple carbs tend to have higher glycemic indices. It's not just candy and sugar that fall into this category; breads and pastas are also full of simple sugars. A simple sugar (or *monosaccharide*) is a type of carbohydrate that cannot be broken down into smaller carbohydrate molecules and is, therefore, rapidly absorbed by the body.

What is added sugar?
Added sugar, also called refined sugar, is any form of sugar or starch that does not exist in nature. While sugar is found naturally in whole foods, it is also often added to processed foods to enhance flavor, or natural sugar may be altered, refined, or processed in some way. It may have been extracted, concentrated, purified, or enzymatically transformed. If it's sweet and was added to food as a crystal, powder, or syrup, it is sugar. There are three simple sugars—sucrose, glucose, and fructose.

The United States Department of Agriculture recently published that Americans consume about 32 teaspoons of added sugar every single day (or 156 pounds every year). Sometimes, we don't even know we are eating it. Added sugar has become our number-one nutritional problem. Researchers at *Nutrition Review* have found that a higher intake of added sugar was associated with poorer diet and a lower intake of nutrients.

And you can trace the beginning of that cycle right to breakfast. Studies show that the more added sugar you eat in the morning, the less healthy food you'll eat all day because foods laced with sugar train our taste buds to want more. But a sugar rush also creates an overflow of insulin in your body as it tries to manage the toxic substance you've just ingested. The body overreacts and pulls too much sugar out of the bloodstream, which can lead you to crash, meaning you will get really tired. So often, people go seeking another sugar rush—one that can't be found from whole foods like carrots and celeries.

The major sources of added sugar in the American diet are:
- sugar-sweetened beverages (37.1%)
- grain-based desserts like cookies or cake (13.7%)
- fruit drinks (8.9%)
- dairy desserts like ice cream (6.1%)
- candy (5.8%)

Many of the foods you buy in the middle section of the grocery store have added sugar, which is very different from the sugar we find in whole foods. Added sugar is used to enhance sweetness and frequently comes from high-fructose corn syrup.

High-fructose corn syrup is a sweetener made from cornstarch that has been chemically altered to separate the fructose from the glucose. This means that when you eat it, the fructose goes right into your liver and turns on fat production. First, it causes fatty liver. Then, it causes prediabetes and type 2 diabetes. It's in many of the processed foods we eat: the average American consumes about forty pounds of high-fructose corn syrup every year, and it is a major contributor to our current epidemics of heart attacks, strokes, obesity, diabetes, cancers, and dementia. And it's loaded with chemicals, including mercury. If this ingredient is in your food, it's food you need to throw out.

[43]

In contrast, whole foods that contain sugar also contain fiber. Fiber is key because it slows down absorption in the intestine, so you don't get a sugar spike when, for instance, you eat an apple. When you eat processed food with added sugar, there's nothing to slow down a blood sugar spike. Experts say it would take six cups of strawberries to equal the blood sugar spike you get from one can of Coke.

Eliminating added sugar, even for as little as nine days, can make huge changes in your health. In contrast, if you go on a binge and start drinking sodas and fruit juices with high-fructose corn syrup, you'll also increase fatty deposits. But there are other ways added sugar contributes to fat in your body. Studies show that a diet made of 18 percent added sugars (the classic American diet) made lab mice lazy and move less.

Candy land

In our family lives and classrooms, we shower our children with love and affection...and sweets—candies, cookies, ice cream, cupcakes, sweet cereals, fruit juices, and sodas. Many traditions in our culture are honored by rewarding youngsters with sugary snacks. Special treats and holidays are built around sugar. A trip to the grocery store ends with a run through the sugar-filled cashier's line. Sugar, in fact, is equated with fun and hominess and good family times. The memories of homemade chocolate-chip cookies are imprinted in their little minds for a lifetime.

However, the American Heart Association recommends children limit daily sugar intake to three or four teaspoons. The World Health Organization suggests limiting sugar consumption to less than 10 percent of total daily calorie intake. Even fruit juice is considered a major contributor to obesity due to its sugar content.

Consider this: at the moment, when our littlest community members' taste buds are being developed, we are linking sugar to their happiest memories and making it difficult for fruits and vegetables to ever compete.

Sugar addiction

Would you give your child a highly addictive narcotic? I didn't think so. And yet, we are indoctrinating our children into a culture of sugar addiction. Once we start eating the sweet stuff, it is

[44]

hard to stop. Sugar is an addictive substance that stimulates the release of neurotransmitters in the brain, such as dopamine and serotonin. Serotonin is a neurotransmitter that elevates your mood. It's not all that different from alcohol, cocaine, and other drugs of abuse. It has been shown, in fact, that it may be even more addictive than cocaine and heroin and that your body becomes dependent upon it.

Then, when you don't eat sugar, you go into withdrawal. Achiness and sluggishness might haunt you. On the other hand, the less sugar you eat, the less you will crave it. Give it up for few days and you'll be over the worst.

Artificial sweeteners

If you thought artificial sweeteners were an acceptable way to satisfy your sweet tooth without gaining weight, think again. Diet soda and the artificial sweeteners do not aid weight loss. Instead, they stimulate the appetite, increase your craving for carbs, and create metabolic havoc in your body, which leads to fat storage and weight gain.

There are five FDA-approved artificial sweeteners—saccharin, acesulfame, aspartame, neotame, and sucralose. Our body responds to these no-calorie or low-calorie sugar replacements in complex ways.

One thing they do is change the way we taste food. Since artificial sweeteners are a lot stronger in taste than table sugar or high-fructose corn syrup, a small amount gives big taste without the calories. The strong flavor of artificial sweeteners may make other foods—like fruits and vegetables—less appealing or flavorless.

They also trick your brain into not associating sweetness with calorie intake, which can lead you to choose sweet food over nutritious foods. Studies show that people who drank more than twenty-one diet sodas per week were twice as likely to become obese as people who didn't drink diet soda.

Artificial sweeteners are as addictive as real sugar. They can also confuse the body's insulin response. Studies of atherosclerosis show that people who drink diet sodas every day are at risk for metabolic syndrome and type 2 diabetes. Despite this, they are added to about six thousand different drinks, snacks, and foods, which make it necessary for you to read the labels on packaged goods.

[45]

Some companies are even trying to add artificial sweeteners to products like milk *and* not have to list it in the ingredients.

When you eat something sweet, your brain releases dopamine, which activates your brain's reward center. Simultaneously, the appetite-regulating hormone leptin is released, which regulates the hunger center in the brain. If you eat something with artificial sweeteners, you confuse your brain, which then overstimulates the hunger center and causes you to eat more.

Sugar content in alcohol

There's not a one-size-fits-all remedy for measuring sugar content when you saddle up to the bar and order a drink. While alcohol can have quite a lot of calories and carbohydrates, it may not always come with lots of sugar. In fact, hard liquors contain almost no sugar—until you start adding in sugary juices and sodas to your cocktails. Beer contains no sugar at all, and a glass of wine contains about a quarter teaspoon of sugar.

While I'm not recommending you start drinking, it is known that modest consumption of alcoholic beverages (ten ounces of wine, twelve ounces of beer, or one and a half ounces of distilled liquor per day) can actually lower your blood sugar. Here's why: Alcohol is metabolized differently than other foods and beverages. Absorbed in the gastrointestinal tract and processed through several pathways, the majority of alcohol is broken down in the liver, which is also where glucose is made. Because of this, alcohol consumption can interfere with the liver's production of glucose and may cause a drop in blood sugar. Alcohol intake can lower blood sugar immediately and up to twelve hours after ingestion.

However, heavy drinkers will eventually experience problems with their insulin, which leads to higher sugar levels. In addition, since our bodies can't store alcohol and must burn it quickly, it will be more difficult to shed body fat when consuming higher amounts of alcohol. When you're considering a drink, remember that adding Coke to rum is like putting seven teaspoons of sugar into your glass. Adding cranberry juice to vodka is the same as heaping in seven and a half teaspoons of sugar. Regardless of sugar content, most drinks contain empty calories, which will contribute to weight gain if consumed in large amounts.

Understanding Your Blood Sugar
There are several different ways to find out how your body is handling sugar, even though there may be no obvious symptoms. Here are some important blood tests to request.

Hemoglobin A1c Test
One way to accurately measure blood sugar level is with a hemoglobin A1c test. The A1c test is a blood test that provides information about a person's average levels of blood glucose, also called blood sugar, over the past three months. It is based on the attachment of glucose to hemoglobin (glycosylation), the protein in red blood cells that carries oxygen. In the body, red blood cells are constantly forming and dying, but typically, they live for about three to four months. Thus, the A1c test reflects the average blood glucose levels over the past three months. The A1c test result is reported as a percentage. The higher the percentage, the higher a person's blood glucose levels have been.

- A normal A1c level is below 5.7 percent. An A1c under 5.7 percent is considered normal.
- An A1c between 5.7 and 6.4 percent is considered prediabetes.
- An A1c equal to or above 6.5 percent is diagnostic for diabetes.

Fasting Blood Glucose Test
A fasting blood glucose test is taken after not eating for at least eight hours. A high level may require a second test a few days later to confirm the reading. If both tests show elevated levels of blood glucose, you may be diagnosed with prediabetes or diabetes.

- For people without diabetes, blood sugar levels after not eating for eight hours ideally should hover around 70 to 85 mg/dl.

[47]

- For some people, 60 may be normal; for others, 90.
- If your level is 126 mg/dl or higher on two separate tests, you have diabetes. If your blood sugar level is 100 to 125 mg/dl, you have borderline diabetes, or prediabetes, due to your body not making enough insulin or not using it properly.

Even if your doctor says you have a slightly elevated blood sugar level (100 to 110 mg/dl) and advises you to watch it, be sure to remind the doc that any elevated fasting blood sugar should be taken seriously.

Fasting Insulin Test
The insulin level in your blood can be measured in the fasting state. While it fluctuates during the day depending on whether or not you have eaten, it should be at nearly zero after you fast for eight or more hours. If it is elevated after fasting, then you may have insulin resistance, an early sign of diabetes (more on this later).

Oral Glucose Tolerance Test
And lastly is a test called *oral glucose tolerance test*, which measures how your body handles sugar. Seventy-five grams of glucose is given by mouth and then your blood sugar level is measured after two hours. This test is often difficult to tolerate and, therefore, is usually not done.

If you're curious about your own sugar level, you could easily invest in an inexpensive glucometer— all diabetics use them. People without diabetes would benefit from having this information too. During the day, levels tend to be at their lowest just before meals.
A new device called continuous glucose monitoring can be used to measure your blood sugar level

[48]

without the fingersticks.
All the above tests together can detect sugar
problems much earlier than the routine fasting blood
sugar.

TIPS:

1. Sugar doesn't only come in candies and ice cream but also in foods we eat every day, like white rice, pasta, bread, dried fruits, ketchup, tomato sauce, barbeque sauce, and salad dressings, so know the sugar content in the foods you eat.
2. Consider not buying any white or brown sugar, agave nectar, or corn syrup. If you have it—dump it.
3. Snack on carrots, celery, fruit, red peppers, roasted almonds, and cherry tomatoes. Get frozen fruit and puree it or eat it whole.
4. Drink lots and lots of water.
5. Maintain your blood sugar level throughout the day by eating regular meals containing complex carbohydrates, lean protein and healthy fats and make sure you get fiber—this will help reduce cravings. Minimize snacking between meals.
6. Don't go out to the grocery store, a restaurant, etc., ravenously hungry. Your cravings will be hard to ignore.
7. If you're tired, stressed, bored, or lonely, try to identify the feeling and do something else besides reaching for sugar as comfort.
8. If you do find yourself reaching for sugar, forgive yourself and start over. Keep trying; don't give up.
9. If you need a sweetener, use stevia.
10. Most toothpaste contains saccharin. Consider changing to toothpaste that does not have saccharin or artificial sweeteners. All foods will taste much sweeter.

Smoking

When you think of the harm smoking does, your mind probably goes straight to the lungs—wheezing, coughing, and cancer. In truth, the real damage from smoking occurs to the circulatory system. While both nicotine and carbon monoxide from cigarette smoke have been studied extensively, it's the smoke itself

[49]

that turns out be much more destructive. Nicotine is highly addictive and has a powerful vasoconstriction effect. The blood vessels become smaller all over the body, reducing blood flow while raising blood pressure and placing more stress on the heart. Carbon monoxide acts independently to reduce the oxygen level in the blood by binding to the hemoglobin—the oxygen-carrying molecule.

Along with nicotine and carbon monoxide, smokers inhale over 7,000 chemicals, 69 known carcinogens, and at least 250 harmful toxins. You wouldn't drink formaldehyde, ammonia, hydrogen cyanide, arsenic, or DDT, would you? But smokers puff away many times on one cigarette. Many of these chemicals come from the burning tobacco leaf. Some of these compounds are chemically active and can cause profound changes within the body.

The most damaging components of tobacco smoke are tar, carbon monoxide, hydrogen cyanide, and oxidizing chemicals including free radicals (rogue electrons) that can damage the heart muscle and blood vessels by causing inflammation in the vessel lining. It's been known for over sixty years that cardiovascular disease (or circulation-related problems) is more common in smokers than nonsmokers and is the most significant cause of smoking-related premature death. In fact, the risk of coronary heart disease is double for men and women who smoke. There are over one billion cigarette smokers in the world. Regrettably, 400,000 Americans die from smoking cigarettes every year.

Secondhand, or *sidestream*, smoke has even higher concentrations of carcinogens than the smoke the smokers themselves inhale. Studies show that it can immediately affect the heart, blood vessels, and circulation in a harmful way. About 54,000 people die every year from secondhand smoke exposure; 48,500 of them die from heart disease. Two out of every five children are exposed to secondhand smoke.

It turns out cigarette smoking tampers with nitric oxide—the molecule that causes blood vessels to relax (vasodilation) allowing the blood to flow easily. The reduction in nitric oxide results in stiffer blood vessels, with less oxygen delivered to the entire body.

Smokers develop major problems with blood flow long before they start to see lung problems. It contributes to heart disease, limb amputation, erectile dysfunction, and stroke. Smokers also have a much higher risk of healing problems, infections, heart attacks, and strokes or developing blood clots with any surgical procedures.

Smoking causes injury inside every blood vessel in the smoker's body. It affects the skin's blood supply and causes wrinkles, early aging, hair loss, and tooth decay; it even affects hearing. Smoking is linked to many kinds of cancer including lung, esophagus, larynx, mouth, throat, kidney, bladder, liver, pancreas, stomach, cervix, colon, rectum, and acute myeloid leukemia. That's right: *smoking increases cancer risk in just about every part of the body.* It ages you; can cause heart disease, stroke, aortic aneurysm, chronic obstructive pulmonary disease, bronchitis, emphysema, diabetes, osteoporosis, age-related macular degeneration, and cataracts; and can worsen asthma.

There are immediate benefits to quitting smoking. After only twenty minutes, your heart rate goes back to normal, and within a day, your blood's carbon monoxide level falls. In just two to three weeks, you will start to lower your odds of having a heart attack. In the long run, you will also lower your chance of getting lung cancer and all other cancers. Quitting smoking is the fastest way to get more oxygen from your lungs to the rest of the body. E-cigarettes and vaping, while less harmful than cigarettes, can still cause nicotine poisoning and contain harmful aerosolized chemicals.

TIPS: *Need help quitting smoking? Because it is such an addictive habit, you may need counseling or hypnotherapy to get over it. The American Cancer Society offers wise advice for getting through the tough days.*

- *The first few days after you quit smoking, spend as much free time as you can in public places where smoking is not allowed. (Libraries, malls, museums, theaters, restaurants without bars, and churches are most often smoke-free.)*
- *Take extra care of yourself. Drink water, eat well, and get enough sleep. This could help you have the energy you might need to handle extra stress.*
- *Don't drink alcohol, coffee, or any other drinks you link with smoking for at least a couple of months. Try something else instead—maybe different types of water or*

[51]

sports drinks. Try to choose drinks that are low or no calorie.

- *If you miss the feeling of having a cigarette in your hand, hold something else—a pencil, a paper clip, a coin, or a marble, for example.*
- *If you miss the feeling of having something in your mouth, try toothpicks, cinnamon sticks, sugarless gum, sugar-free lollipops, or celery. Some people chew on a straw or stir stick.*
- *Avoid temptation—stay away from activities, people, and places you link with smoking.*
- *Create new habits and a nonsmoking environment around you.*
- *Get ready to face future situations or crises that might make you want to smoke again and think of all the important reasons you've decided to quit. To remind yourself of these reasons, put a picture of the people who are the most important to you somewhere you see it every day or keep one handy on your phone.*
- *Take deep breaths to relax. Picture your lungs filling with fresh, clean air.*
- *Remember your goal and the fact that the urge to smoke will lessen over time.*
- *Think about how awesome it is that you're quitting smoking and getting healthy. If you start to weaken, remember your goal. Remember that quitting is a learning process. Be patient with yourself.*
- *Brush your teeth and enjoy that fresh taste.*
- *Exercise in short bursts. Try alternately tensing and relaxing muscles, push-ups, lunges, walking up the stairs, or touching your toes.*
- *Call a friend, family member, or a stop-smoking help line when you need extra help or support.*
- *Above all, reward yourself for doing your best. Give yourself rewards often if that's what it takes to keep going. Plan to do something fun.*

Processed Food

The processed food sector is a multi-billion-dollar industry in the United States alone. No trip to an American supermarket would be complete without meandering through aisle upon aisle of every conceivable item of processed food—microwaveable meals, "instant" foods, condiments, cheese, energy bars—the list goes on and on. It's no surprise then, that huge companies like General Mills and Mondelez hire scores of food scientists to tinker with color, flavor, smell, and texture to make the food look and taste better, extend shelf life, cut costs, and ensure you buy them again and again. Some foods have been so processed and stripped of most of their natural nutrients that they aren't really food at all. These chemicals, however, are causing serious harm to your body.

For the most part, our bodies do not recognize the chemicals in processed food, many of which are toxic to our blood vessels and cells, causing free radical formation and inflammation. Many of the foods also contain added sugar or sugar substitutes, both of which also affect the circulatory system.

So, while you're shopping for food, pay close attention and beware of the following eight ingredients:

1. Trans Fats (Partially Hydrogenated Oil)

Adding hydrogen to liquid vegetable oil will yield solid fat and becomes partially hydrogenated oil or trans fat. Trans fat is difficult for the body to dissolve, and this is the worst type of fat you can consume. This man-made fat is different from naturally occurring trans fat—chemically altered trans fats contributes to heart disease, diabetes, inflammation, and arterial stiffness. Companies use hydrogenated trans fats to stabilize flavor and extend shelf life of foods. There is a dizzying array of foods that contain trans fats, including margarine, vegetable shortening, baked goods, (particularly those with frosting), cereals, coffee creamer, fried fast foods, and frozen pizza.

2. Preservatives

BHA and BHT (Butylated Hydroxyanisole and Butylated Hydroxytoluene):

These are antioxidant preservatives used in everything from potato chips to chewing gum and cereals to keep them from getting spoiled. But contrary to what you may think about antioxidants as being healthy, these specific ones can potentially cause cancer. The FDA allows them and placed them in a category of Generally Recognized As Safe (GRAS). However, the National Toxicology Program of the Department of Health and Human Services determined that BHA was *"reasonably anticipated to be a human carcinogen based on sufficient evidence of carcinogenicity from studies in experimental animals."* Despite the conflicting studies with regards to carcinogenic effects of BHT, it's been banned in several countries (note that BHT is also used in makeup). Although the health effects of these preservatives on humans are unclear at this point, staying away from preservatives altogether is a better and safer choice.

Sodium Nitrate and Sodium Nitrite:

Adding pink and red color to deli meats, hot dogs, bacon, and even certain types of fish makes them more palatable. But sodium nitrate and sodium nitrite can form nitrosamine in the stomach, which can increase the risk of cancer. Sodium nitrate and nitrite are preservatives and color fixatives mostly found in processed meats like hot dogs, bacon, ham, and cold cuts. They have been linked to colorectal cancer; the World Health Organization recently equated the consumption of processed meats to be as harmful as cigarette smoking. Stick to natural grass-fed or organic meats.

Propyl Gallate:

Even fats and oils can spoil, so to prevent that from happening, companies add propyl gallate to BHA and BHT. It can cause allergic reaction in humans and has been shown to cause cancer in animal studies. It can be found in things like vegetable oil, potato sticks, packaged meat products, chewing gum, and even some chicken soup broth.

Sodium Benzoate and Benzoic Acid:

Microorganisms tend to grow in acidic products after they sit around for a while—think sauerkraut, jellies, jams, hot sauces, and soda. That's where sodium benzoate and benzoic acid come into to play, which are used by companies to slow or stop the growth of those organisms. They are found in very small amounts in foods and generally considered safe. These two are naturally occurring acids and only bother people with allergies. But when sodium benzoate is combined with ascorbic acid (a.k.a. vitamin C), it can form small amounts of benzene, a chemical that causes leukemia and other blood cancers. Higher amounts of benzene have been found in soft drinks, with some brands exceeding safe limits, according to FDA reports.

3. Sweeteners
High Fructose Corn Syrup (HFCS):

High fructose corn syrup is an artificial sugar made from genetically modified corn. It is half-glucose and half-fructose. While it is chemically similar to table sugar (sucrose), it is cheaper and highly processed form of glucose converted into fructose. The other problem is that it is added to almost every packaged food and sauce, increasing your sugar intake. Some food companies list HFCS as *natural sweetener*. Consumption of HFCS has been linked to high blood pressure, increased risk for diabetes, fatty liver, obesity, and other metabolic disorders. It also causes the formation of free radicals and inflammation, leading to increased cancer.

Artificial Sweeteners (aspartame, sucralose, acesulfame, neotame, saccharin):

Since these satisfy your sweet tooth with no calories, many consider them safe alternatives to sugar. But studies have shown that they lead to increased risk of diabetes, obesity, and metabolic syndrome.

4. Artificial and Natural Flavoring
Natural and artificial flavoring is done to entice you into eating more. The natural flavoring comes from edible source while artificial from inedible. They are both made from chemicals. Common artificial flavors like caramel can cause health issues that include genetic defects and cancer. Don't think just because its "natural" that it is safe. Some natural flavors can contain traces of cyanide and can be more dangerous than artificial flavors. Ironically, artificial flavors also go through more rigorous safety guidelines.

[55]

5. Flour Improver

Walk through the bread aisle of any supermarket in the United States and you're more than likely to find a wide array of bread products containing bromated flour—that is, flour containing potassium bromate, or simply bromate. Bread companies use oxidizing agent in the flour to strengthen the dough, making breads and rolls soft, elastic, and voluminous with that appealing white color. But as tasty as the bread may be, the International Agency for Research on Cancer determined in 1999 that potassium bromate was "possibly carcinogenic to humans" based on "sufficient evidence in experimental animals."

Recognizing the destructive quality of this chemical in food, most industrialized countries have banned this chemical—except for the United States. Despite the overwhelming evidence that bromate causes inflammation and free radicals and DNA damage, it's still being used in many of the breads, crackers, and baked goods sitting on our grocery shelves.

6. Food Coloring

Color is important to how we experience food. But what's scary is that food dyes find their way into many foods, especially children's foods, like boxed mac and cheese or fruit juice. The FDA puts it this way: "Without color additives, colas wouldn't be brown, margarine wouldn't be yellow, and mint ice cream wouldn't be green. Color additives are now recognized as an important part of practically all processed foods we eat." It's shocking that we consume nearly 17.8 million pounds of artificial food dyes every year. While originally made from coal tar, these additives now can be made from petroleum, among other things. Many food dyes have been banned throughout the world, but many dangerous ones still remain, and the FDA has yet to ban them. The most widely used food dye Red #40, which has been linked to tumors in mice and hyperactivity in children. Red #3 has been shown to cause cancer in animals, while Yellow #5 and #6 may cause thyroid and kidney tumors, lymphocytic lymphomas, and especially chromosomal damage. Natural food coloring, such as carotenoids, chlorophyll, anthocyanin (found in many blue or purple fruits and vegetables, like blueberries and eggplant), and turmeric, while safer also has shorter shelf life and therefore is much more expensive. To cut costs, food manufacturers resort to using the cheaper chemical color additives.

7. Flavor Enhancer (MSG)

Monosodium Glutamate (MSG) is one of the most widely used food additives. It's added as a food enhancer that intensifies flavor by heightening your taste buds; it provides a certain umami that's hard to replicate naturally (which is why that ramen tastes so good!). But MSG is a nerve stimulant and can damage your brain cells. It's often added to many processed foods like diet beverages, canned foods, instant soup, packaged sausages, hot dogs, salad dressings, and even some packaged vegetarian foods. It's also a commonly used ingredient in Asian cuisine. This additive is listed under many different names, but no matter what it's called, it contributes to obesity, type 2 diabetes, metabolic syndrome, and inflammation.

8. Advanced Glycation End Products (AGEs)

This one is a little trickier. AGEs are related to the way food is prepared—at home and in factories. Explaining AGEs requires a crash course in chemical research history. In prewar 1912, a young French physician and chemist named Louis Camille Maillard was curious about the chemical reaction between nutrient sugars (such as glucose and fructose) and amino acids, the building blocks of proteins.

When Maillard heated a water-based solution of sugars and amino acids for a few hours, they turned a yellow-brown color—the result of a series of reactions that produced a harmful concoction of products. What the Frenchman had discovered were important chemical reactions that are now referred to as the *Maillard reaction* with AGEs as their end product.

AGEs are implicated in the development or exacerbation of a whole host of diseases associated with aging—type 2 diabetes, atherosclerosis, cardiovascular disease, Alzheimer's and other dementias, cataracts, retinal dysfunction, kidney failure, nerve damage, arthritis, and cancer.

Glycation, the first step in his reaction, is when a sugar molecule binds to an amino acid in a protein. It happens in our body naturally, but we get a lot more of it from much of the delicious food

[57]

we eat—food that is put through certain heating methods. Chefs love glycation because it produces food that tastes good. Companies that produce processed food use glycation for the coloring or in the way the foods are made. Browning the food you cook by roasting, baking, grilling, frying, sautéing, or broiling creates AGEs. Boiling or steaming meats and vegetables is better, or slow cooking meats so they don't get that crunchy, charred layer on the outside.

> **TIPS:** *Real food is generally found around the edges of the grocery store—the produce, meat, and dairy sections. Try to stay out of the middle of the store; that's where most of the processed food is. Read the label. Multiple ingredients should raise a red flag. Don't eat food with ingredients you don't recognize.*
> *Colors matter, as in the colors of a rainbow. Naturally occurring red, orange, yellow, blue, and purple are usually signs of healthy food. Brown is a red flag for advanced glycation end products. Try to avoid over browning or burning food.*

Stress

Neuroscientists have made startling discoveries about stress in the past two decades, and one of the biggest revelations is that your brain is wired to keep you stressed. Basically, fears and wants sustain your stress level. A few million years ago, our hunter-and-gatherer ancestors survived by recognizing threats and flaws in dangerous environments. As the body prepared for battle, cortisol and adrenaline would flood the bloodstream, and blood sugars and cholesterol levels would spike. The heart would start pumping harder, and blood pressure would rise. Breathing became stronger and quicker to get more oxygen into the body. In the wake of all that, blood consistency would become stickier, fat molecules wouldn't be cleared out as quickly, and there was thickening in the blood vessel wall, weakening of immune function and slowing of digestion.

It still happens that way today. Our body produces a stress hormone called cortisol, which acts as a conductor during the body's orchestrated reaction to stress. During stress, cortisol directs blood sugar levels, fat, protein and carbohydrate metabolism, immune responses, anti-inflammatory actions, blood pressure, and heart and blood vessel tone, and it also activates the central nervous system.

[58]

But nowadays, we don't need the same physical reaction because we rarely face the kind of physical threats our ancestors did. Once the stress reaction starts, the body often fails to take note that we're no longer in danger, and so the stress continues to surge.

During calm days, cortisol levels peak in our body at 8:00 a.m. and reach their lowest at 4:00 a.m. Our health depends on the adrenal glands secreting cortisol, but also on the cortisol returning to normal levels after a stressful event. Too much cortisol can lead to weight gain and blood vessel injury.

As survival mode sets in during stress, cortisol moves fat from healthy areas of the body into your midsection. This is the main reason why stress increases visceral fat (the unhealthy fat deep inside your belly) and encourages weight gain and inflammation.

Whether it's because you are running from a saber-toothed tiger or because you are worried about a project due at work, stress causes the same physiological reaction. But seldom do modern-day causes of stress require the same physical feats of survival or fight-or-flight response that stressors called for a few million years ago. Lots of events and changes—such as relationship issues, money problems, or difficult decisions—can kick in your stress reactions. Traumatic events, the deaths of loved ones, natural disasters, or physical and mental traumas can trigger stress impulses.

Think of those stress impulses like you would a split personality. On one hand, stress is the helpful friend causing hormones to surge through the body, critical for our survival. But the other side of stress is sinister, creating chaos in our chemistry that leads to restlessness, anxiety, emptiness, malaise, an inability to focus, insomnia, fatigue, irritability, and apathy.

Stress can cause hair loss and weight gain. It may cause rashes, headaches, nausea, and diarrhea. The immune system gets blunted which makes it harder to recover from viruses, and wounds take longer to heal. Your vision may change. You may even have difficulty breathing. During stress, your pupils may dilate as you prepare to stare down your foe. Your body gets hungry in anticipation of famine.

The body's stress reactions are hardwired for long-ago days. While the brain-body relationship is complicated, and scientists are not quite certain why stress manifests differently in different people, they are sure that stress affects circulation.

So how do we reduce stress, a mental and physiological reaction that has been in place for millions of years? After all, threats and unpleasant events capture our attention more than happy events do, don't they? It's about being more flexible with our interpretations of events, training our minds to become quiet and more focused, compassionate, nonjudgmental, accepting, and forgiving. Surprisingly, doing this will help calm our brains by disrupting a continuous stress response that can be very damaging to our bodies.

Here's a study to ponder: At Wayne State University in Detroit, researchers looked at 230 pictures of Major League Baseball players from 1952 and found that the players with the biggest smiles lived 79.9 years versus their straight-faced peers who lived 72.9 years. Smiling and laughing leads to a reduction in blood pressure, lower blood sugar, a dulling of pain and stress, and anxiety alleviation.

Yoga is recommended by the American Heart Association for people healing from heart attacks or cardiac arrest. It has calming effects that lower your blood pressure after the very first practice. After twelve weeks, blood pressure, cholesterol, and triglycerides decline further. Meditation is also a beneficial mind-body relaxer. By focusing on not actively thinking, meditation can help us gain new perspective and manage symptoms of anxiety, heart disease, high blood pressure, and associated illnesses.

From living in the present to feeling grateful for small moments, and from meditation and yoga to praying and even smiling, you can reduce stress by exploring the mind-body connection.

TIPS: Any kind of physical activity—even a brisk twenty-minute walk—can have the same calming effect as a mild tranquilizer. Yoga, a mind-body practice that employs physical poses, controlled breathing, and meditation, can be especially helpful. It can lower your blood pressure and heart rate. Physical activity will also reduce the sugar in your bloodstream that has built up from stressful situations. It tricks your body into believing that you are escaping stress. For stress relief, you can reboot during the day by meditating. Take a short break to meditate and combine it with breathing techniques aimed at calming you down—like pushing a reset button.

Also, sleep deprivation is a chronic stressor that contributes to weight gain. Sleeping seven to nine hours a day decreases cortisol level and lowers stress.

Cell

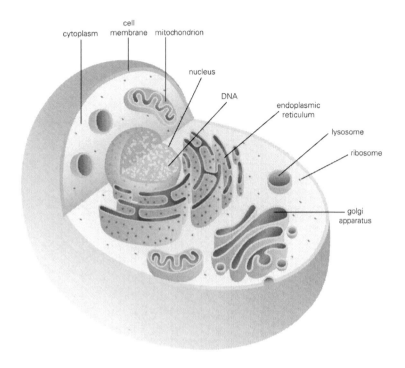

Cell Membrane

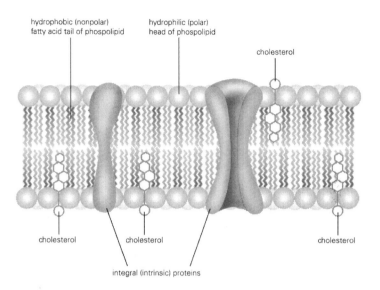

hydrophobic (nonpolar)
fatty acid tail of phospolipid

hydrophilic (polar)
head of phospolipid

cholesterol

cholesterol

cholesterol

cholesterol

integral (intrinsic) proteins

Capillary

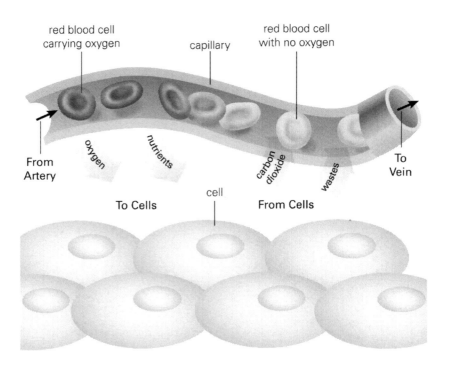

red blood cell
carrying oxygen

capillary

red blood cell
with no oxygen

oxygen

nutrients

carbon
dioxide

wastes

From
Artery

To
Vein

To Cells

cell

From Cells

Plaque Rupture

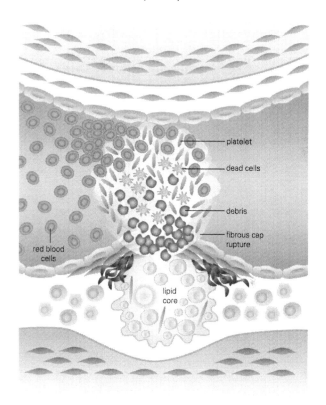

platelet

dead cells

debris

fibrous cap rupture

red blood cells

lipid core

Inflammation

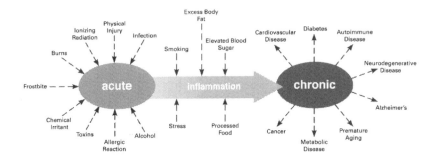

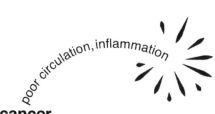

poor circulation, inflammation

cancer

diet

vascular disease

heart disease

hemoglobin A1c **blindness**

high blood sugar metabolic syndrome

pancreas **obesity** **type 2** **exercise** **insulin**

free radicals

diabetes

finger stick mitochondria type 1

refined carbohydrate **glucometer** **foot ulcers** **pre diabetes**

b-cells metformin

insulin resistance glucose tolerance test

hyperglycemia

insulin shots

Blue Zone

LOMA, LINDA UNITED STATES

HEALTHY SOCIAL CIRCLE

EAT NUTS

WHOLE GRAINS

HIGH SOY CONSUMPTION

CULTURALLY ISOLATED

FAMILY

NO SMOKING

NO ALCOHOL

PLANT-BASED DIET

FAITH

CONSTANT MODERATE PHYSICAL ACTIVITY

SOCIAL ENGAGEMENT

FAVA BEANS

LEGUMES

NO "TIME URGENCY"

HIGH POLYPHENOL WINE

EMPOWERED WOMEN

LIKEABILITY

SUNSHINE

TURMERIC

GARDENING

SARDINIA, ITALY

OKINAWA, JAPAN

Mediterranean Diet

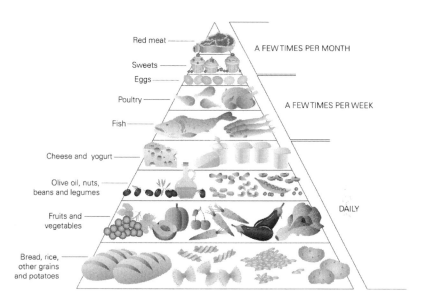

Red meat — A FEW TIMES PER MONTH

Sweets —

Eggs —

Poultry — A FEW TIMES PER WEEK

Fish —

Cheese and yogurt —

Olive oil, nuts, beans and legumes —

Fruits and vegetables — DAILY

Bread, rice, other grains and potatoes —

Chapter 4: Diseases of Our Circulation

As your circulatory system gets stiff and slow from the influences previously discussed, it starts to short circuit. Nearly all diseases begin with blood vessels that can't do their job, leading to slowed blood delivery. This is, of course, a simplified statement of many complex issues, but the truth is that if you mess up your blood vessels with bad living, disease will follow. After all, when your blood can't get life-sustaining oxygen and nutrients to tissues, cells will struggle to survive and organs will malfunction. Those diseases aren't isolated and they stem from our bodies' protective response against relentless assaults.

Below are the major maladies that happen inside your circulatory system when you don't treat it well:

High Blood Pressure

Most people develop hypertension during their fifties and sixties as a result of years of injury to their blood vessels. When your blood vessels are injured by sugar, stress, chemicals in processed foods, being overweight, smoking, and inflammation, they begin to lose flexibility. They become stiff, rigid pipes, and blood has more difficulty flowing through them. Now the heart is forced to pump harder to push the same amount of blood, further elevating blood pressure and amplifying a vicious cycle of blood vessel damage.

Half of Americans over the age of sixty have high blood pressure, called *hypertension*, and a mere 50 percent of those have gotten it successfully under control. Some people never get diagnosed; others refuse medication or aren't taking enough to bring the blood pressure down.

To find out if your blood pressure is too high, you have to understand the fraction-like number the doctor gives you when it is taken. The top number refers to the amount of pressure in your arteries during contraction of your heart muscle, and we call this *systolic pressure*. The bottom number refers to the pressure when your heart muscle relaxes; this is called *diastolic pressure*. Blood pressure relates directly to your arteries' ability to expand (*vasodilation*) and contract (*vasoconstriction*). Blood pressure readings are expressed as millimeters of mercury, which is abbreviated as *mm Hg*.

[70]

Normal pressure is less than 120/80 mmHg. If your blood pressure is higher than that, you have hypertension. The heart muscle ends up working harder to overcome the increased pressure of the blood pushing back at it, and this stresses the heart. Eventually, the heart muscle gets thicker and requires more oxygen to do the same job, which is why heart attacks occur more frequently in people with high blood pressure. Even short periods of elevated pressure can lead to thickening in the arteries, inflamed blood vessels, and atherosclerosis. High blood pressure can pound against your blood vessel walls, impairing their ability to be flexible. Fragile capillaries may stop working temporarily, to protect themselves from the injuring force of elevated pressure. When capillaries shut down, this further impedes the blood flow. Since oxygen exchange occurs in the teeniest capillaries, cells get less oxygen if blood pressure remains high for an extended period of time.

There are no symptoms for high blood pressure—it's called the "silent killer." Even if your blood pressure only goes up at a doctor's office, a.k.a. white coat syndrome, injury to your blood vessel is still occurring. Beyond heart attacks and strokes, it can damage kidneys, limbs, and eyes. If you have it, and your doctor prescribes medication, it is imperative that you take it and try to get your blood pressure under control. Here are some alarming statistics:

Blood pressure higher than 140/90 is seen in:
- 69% of people who have their first heart attack
- 77% of people who have their first stroke
- 74% of people who have congestive heart failure[6]

If you're one of the millions of people with uncontrolled hypertension, your arteries may be paying the price. Normalizing your blood pressure quickly is critical for your blood vessel health. Medication will help control symptoms, but changing your lifestyle is the only way to cure high blood pressure.

TIPS: 1. Replace salt with other spices. Salt raises the amount of sodium in your bloodstream, distorts the delicate balance of your blood content, and increases water retention by the kidneys. The result is higher blood pressure due to the extra fluid and injury to the blood vessels in the kidneys.

[71]

2. Try not to drink more than three alcoholic drinks in one sitting because it can raise your blood pressure to unhealthy levels. One drink is considered 12 ounces of beer, 5 ounces of wine, or 1.5 ounces of eighty-proof distilled spirits. Consume moderate amounts.

3. A waist measurement greater than thirty-five inches for women and forty inches for men can also stress larger blood vessels and cause high blood pressure.

4. Nicotine is a vasoconstrictor. It causes blood vessels to shrink and tighten up, which causes blood pressure to rise.

5. Increasing physical activity will lower your blood pressure.

6. If you need medication to control your blood pressure, a class of medicine called ACE inhibitors (angiotensin converting enzyme) is very effective. Lisinopril is an ACE inhibitor that works by relaxing blood vessels (even the smallest ones) and delivering more oxygen to cells.

Diabetes

The ultimate disease of our circulatory system—diabetes—develops when our blood sugar level gets too high. It causes problems in our blood vessels that can put us at risk for heart attacks, strokes, blindness, kidney failure, neuropathy, and a whole host of other blood-vessel-related illnesses.

To understand diabetes, let's first look inside beta cells, located in the pancreas, where insulin is made and stored. For our body to function properly, we need to convert sugar—our fuel—from food into energy. Insulin is the hormone responsible for regulating sugar levels in the blood. As blood sugar levels rise, beta cells respond quickly by secreting some of their stored insulin, while simultaneously producing more of the hormone. The main role of insulin is to help deliver sugar to the cells to be used for energy. In diabetics, either there's not an adequate amount of insulin being produced, or there's enough but it is unable to do its job adequately.

In addition to keeping our blood sugar levels under control, insulin can also store extra sugar as fat if it's not needed for energy. If we eat a Nutella crepe, our blood sugar will rise whether we are diabetic or not. Promptly, our insulin will be released to deal with the spike in our blood sugar. Any sugar that is not burned as energy or stored as glycogen gets turned into fat, which is also the job of insulin; it's known as the fat-storing hormone. That's why we can gain more body fat by eating a high-carb fat-free dessert than from eating a fat-laden steak. Insulin can tell our body to go from fat-burning (lipolysis) to fat-storage mode (lipogenesis).

Long before a person develops diabetes, he or she will experience problems metabolizing sugar. The first problem is insulin resistance, which is at epidemic levels in the United States and most of the developed world today. Insulin resistance (IR) is the stepping-stone to diabetes, and diabetes is the third leading cause of death in our country[7].

Besides making it difficult for us to lose weight and causing our guts to protrude, insulin resistance results in fatty liver, creates lipid disorder (cholesterol imbalance), and leads to massive blood vessel damage. When we have IR, our muscles and tissues don't hear or respond to insulin's knock to open the cell door. Sugar gets left outside. The pancreas keeps making insulin—more than it needs—and the body isn't able to use it. Excess sugar builds up in the bloodstream, which makes us vulnerable to developing prediabetes, type 2 diabetes, and, most importantly, diseased blood vessels.

If you have a hard time losing abdominal fat, are craving sweets and refined carbohydrates on a daily basis or get shaky when you go without food for several hours, you may have insulin resistance. If you have a family history of diabetes or have excess abdominal fat, you may be prone to insulin resistance. Just as women with a waist circumference greater than thirty-five inches and men with a waist circumference greater than forty inches have an increased risk of high blood pressure, they also have an increased risk for diabetes. If you have any of these symptoms, you may be one of the eighty-six million Americans who are considered prediabetic. Unfortunately, people with this issue may not even know it, and they are certainly not being treated for it.

Prediabetes means that your blood sugar level is higher than normal but not yet high enough to be classified as type 2 diabetes. Already, your body is having difficulty processing sugar—sugar level begins to rise in your bloodstream. Without intervention, prediabetes is likely to become type 2 diabetes in ten years or less. If you have prediabetes, the long-term damage of diabetes—especially to your heart and circulatory system—may already be starting. If you

[73]

change your diet and begin to exercise, you can stop it from progressing to diabetes. And you'd be wise to do so—studies show that if your blood sugar is at prediabetes levels, you have a 59 percent increased chance of cardiovascular disease (CVD) compared to people who have normal blood sugar levels. A Harvard study of nondiabetics with hemoglobin A1c of higher than 5.5, showed an elevated risk for cardiovascular disease[8].

Risk factors for diabetes include those mentioned above as well as being over forty-five, eating a high-sugar diet, having high blood pressure, and suffering from cardiovascular disease. You may also be at risk if you are inactive, have a history of polycystic ovarian syndrome or gestational diabetes, or have a whacky cholesterol profile. If any of these describes you, you should be screened for diabetes. This includes having blood tests for fasting blood sugar, hemoglobin A1c, LP-IR (lipoprotein-insulin resistance test), and fasting insulin level. These tests will tip you off to trouble brewing in the circulatory system.

It is estimated that twenty-nine million people in the United States have diabetes, and that 28 percent of those are undiagnosed. Type 1 diabetes is usually diagnosed in children and young adults and only occurs in 5 to 10 percent of people with diabetes. In type 1 diabetes, the pancreas cannot make any insulin. Doctors don't know what causes type 1—perhaps genetics or exposure to certain viruses or environmental factors (that injure the beta cells). It's type 2 that affects the majority of people—either your body isn't making enough insulin, or it can't use it efficiently to get glucose into the cells. Even in type 2 diabetics, the pancreas can burn out and require insulin injections.

While there's a litany of risk factors, you do in fact have some control over whether you'll get it or if you can be cured. One thing you can control is having too much body fat. Why does excess fat increase your risk for type 2 diabetes? Extra body fat, especially around the middle, creates insulin resistance. Researchers think that being overweight stresses the insides of individual cells. Gaining as little as ten pounds over fifteen years can double your insulin resistance! At present, more than 78.6 million adult Americans are considered obese (that's more than *one-third*), and obese people are *seven* times more likely to develop diabetes than those with a healthy weight.

[74]

Regular exercise and a change in eating will normalize your sugar level and, very likely, result in weight loss. Even a small amount of weight loss can have a big impact on your insulin sensitivity.

The effects of diabetes on blood vessels are a magnified version of the effects that sugar (glucose) itself can have. Whether you're a diabetic or a prediabetic, or you experience sugar spikes an hour or so after a meal, your blood vessels' lining take a beating. Sticky sugar gloms on to everything in your blood and can jam up the vessels' ability to expand. High blood sugar promotes free radical formation and inflammation, which eventually lead to what we've already spelled out as bad news—atherosclerosis. But it doesn't stop there. High blood sugar levels also destroy small vessels by thickening capillary walls and even interfering with new vessel growth. Additionally, elevated insulin will unleash inflammatory messengers that can wreck our blood vessels. There is a tsunami effect on our entire circulatory system, culminating in heart disease, stroke, kidney disease, loss of vision, peripheral vascular disease, wound healing issues, infections, loss of limbs, and cancer. It also affects nerves. More than half of diabetics suffer from neuropathy, which causes debilitating problem in the legs and the feet. The shooting pain and pins-and-needles sensations that sufferers experience are due to damaged nerves not getting enough oxygen.

TIP: Observing a daily routine of healthy eating, tracking refined carbohydrates, and exercising is the cornerstone in getting your blood sugar under control. Sugar testing is also important. Medication such as metformin maybe needed to avoid, delay the onset or treat diabetes. If you have a sugar problem but are not yet a diabetic, you can still experience all the circulation problems that come with diabetes. Strict blood sugar control should be number-one priority for everyone.

Following are the blood tests to look for excess sugar in your blood: (I know you read this before, but it's worth reviewing again.)

Hemoglobin A1c Test

The A1c test is a blood test that provides information about a person's average levels of blood sugar over the past three months. It is based on the attachment of glucose to hemoglobin (glycosylation), the protein in red blood cells that carries oxygen. Since red blood cells live for about three to four months, the A1c test reflects your average blood sugar level over the past three months.

-A normal A1c level is below 5.7 percent, although multiple studies show a higher risk for cardiovascular disease when it is above 5.5.

-An A1c between 5.7 and 6.4 percent is considered prediabetes.

-An A1c equal to or above 6.5 percent is diagnostic for diabetes.

Fasting Blood Glucose Test

A fasting blood glucose test is taken after not eating for at least eight hours. A high level may require a second test a few days later to confirm the reading.

-For people without diabetes, blood sugar levels after not eating for eight hours ideally should hover around 70 to 85 mg/dl.

-For some people, 60 may be normal; for others, 90.

-The current acceptable level is below 100, but recent studies indicate that a level of 91 to 99 is associated with increased risk for diabetes.

-If your level is 126 mg/dl or higher on two separate tests, you have diabetes. If your blood sugar level is 100 to 125 mg/dl, you have borderline diabetes, or prediabetes.

Fasting Insulin Test

The insulin level in your blood can be measured in the fasting state. While it fluctuates during the day depending on whether or not you have eaten, it should be at nearly zero after you fast for eight or more hours. If it is elevated after fasting, then you may have insulin resistance, an early sign of diabetes.

[76]

LP-IR Score
This test looks at all the lipoproteins (LDL, HDL, VLDL)
using a nuclear magnetic resonance (NMR) spectroscopy.
Since sugar and lipid metabolism are closely linked—looking
at the size and concentration of the lipoproteins can
determine the risk for insulin resistance. LP-IR score is used
as an early predictor for diabetes.

Oral Glucose Tolerance Test
This measures how your body processes sugar. Seventy-five
grams of glucose is given by mouth and then your blood
sugar level is measured after two hours. It is done at the
doctor's office.

Blood Glucose Meter Test
This is a portable blood sugar test. Using an inexpensive
glucometer (about $20), you can check your blood glucose at
any time. During the day, levels tend to be at their lowest just
before meals.
All the above tests together can detect sugar problems much
earlier than the routine fasting blood sugar test.

Continuous Glucose Monitoring
A new tech device that is placed on your upper arm will
measure your blood sugar continuously. You can use a
portable monitor or a smartphone to see the results.
Currently Dexcom and Abbott Libre System are available.

Obesity

Obesity is one of the most pervasive, chronic diseases and a leading cause of death and sickness in the United States. It puts tremendous pressure on our healthcare system in terms of both cost and resources.

Excess adipose tissue is the main hallmark of obesity. It sends elevated levels of free fatty acids into the blood, triggering inflammation and stiffening blood vessels. Reactive changes occur in the kidney and the nervous system, adversely affecting arteries and elevating blood pressure. Being obese also predisposes one to insulin resistance, prediabetes, and type 2 diabetes. It might surprise you to know that a fat cell is much more than a storage depot—it's actually an endocrine organ that secretes hormones. Fat cells have an ideal size, but as they enlarge, they start to secrete all sorts of proinflammatory products into the body, adding to the ongoing inflammation.

The fastest way to add fat to your body is by eating—and the fastest way to become obese (defined by your body mass index or BMI) is to overeat. Your brain responds to triggers like smell, taste, texture, and temperature in food as well as your own memories and emotions as it guides you to begin or stop eating. But scientists have also discovered two important hormones secreted by fat that play major roles in obesity: adiponectin and leptin.

Adiponectin promotes both sugar and fat metabolism, but as people gain weight, adiponectin levels drop. As inflammation and insulin resistance set in the blood vessels are the first to be affected.

Leptin's role is to inhibit hunger by controlling appetite in the brain's hypothalamus. As people gain weight, leptin levels increase, the body becomes resistant to leptin and the brain doesn't send the signals of satiety after eating. The more weight you gain, the harder it is to feel full.

A whopping 69 percent of American adults are considered obese or to be carrying excess weight. Being obese puts you at risk for more than thirty chronic diseases—type 2 diabetes, hypertension, gallstones, heart disease, fatty liver disease, sleep apnea, GERD, stress incontinence, heart failure, degenerative joint disease, birth defects, miscarriages, asthma and other respiratory conditions, and numerous cancers. Many of these can trace their beginnings directly back to stiff blood vessels.

For instance, one of the most reliable predictors of heart disease and atherosclerosis is abdominal obesity. Let's take a closer look at that belly fat because it falls into two categories: visceral and subcutaneous. Visceral fat is found deep down in your belly, surrounding your organs (like fatty liver). It's the most dangerous kind and the one that links directly to heart disease. In excess it can even strangle an organ. Chronic stress, which causes increased cortisol production, promotes visceral fat accumulation. Some people with weight gain are genetically predisposed to store more of this dangerous visceral fat as opposed to the subcutaneous fat, which is found just below the skin. (CT scan of the abdomen is an effective method to measure visceral fat).

Since 1980, we have effectively swapped smoking for obesity. The obesity rate in the United States has nearly tripled while cigarette smoking has been halved. This has been a windfall for the food and pharmaceutical industries, as they have developed multiple drugs targeting high blood pressure, diabetes, weight reduction, digestive problems, back and joint issues, and sleep apnea. These same food companies who have made us fat are now soliciting dieters with low-carb, low-fat, low-cal, sugar-free, "healthy" options; diet supplements; and weight-reduction meal plans.

Because we think of obesity as a disease, we have accepted it as part of our lives and often believe we can't control it. Smoking, on the other hand, is considered a bad habit that we can overcome. Keep in mind that with obesity, we still get all the circulation-related problems in our body but in more insidious ways.

To know if you're obese, you'll need to measure your body mass index (BMI). BMI is a mathematical calculation involving height and weight. It is calculated by dividing a person's body weight in kilograms by their height in meters squared (weight [kg] height $[m]^2$) or by using the conversion with pounds (lbs.) and inches (in.) squared as shown below. This number can be misleading, however, for very muscular people or for pregnant or lactating women.

[Weight (lbs.) ÷ height (in.)^2] x 704.5 = BMI
The BMI cutoffs are:

Below 18.5	Underweight
18.5–24.9	Normal weight
24.5–29.9	Overweight
30 and greater	Obese
40 and greater	Morbid or extreme obesity

You should also be aware of your waist circumference, which measures your abdominal fat. As mentioned a few times above, excess abdominal fat, when out of proportion to total body fat, is considered a major risk factor for heart disease (as well as high blood pressure and diabetes).

TIPS: Two strategies for fighting obesity are moving and eating. The first one can be pretty simple. Stand up. Sitting poses a clear and present danger to your health. Too much of it, even if you are doing aerobic exercise, is associated with higher rates of obesity. It also causes physiological damage because your blood flow slows down, calorie-burning rate drops immediately, your blood sugar rises, and your insulin level goes up. Your body goes into fat-storage mode and you will gain weight. Recently, prolonged sitting has been shown to be even worse than smoking! Ninety percent of energy expended in all forms of physical activity occurs during standing and not while exercising. Whether you exercise five times a week or not, you still need to limit all the sitting time. Here are some advices on eating:

- *Use utensils that help you to be more precise about what you pick up to eat.*
- *Limit eating handheld food like hamburgers, pizza, and sandwiches—it's hard to judge how much you are eating.*
- *Always exercise portion control.*
- *Choose food quality over quantity.*
- *Beware of calorie counting because all foods are not created equal. Some foods, such as processed and refined carbs, can add to obesity risk, while complex carbs are able to be burned quickly.*
- *Eat slower.*
- *Do not make children eat everything on their plates.*
- *Stop expecting excessive amounts of food on certain holidays and when out at restaurants. Change your mindset—smaller portions are better.*
- *As you age, your metabolism slows, and you move less; therefore, you need to eat less.*
- *Be careful of consuming sweetened beverages.*
- *Desserts should not always be part of a meal.*
- *Drink plenty of water!*

Heart Disease

A prominent heart surgeon who regularly looks inside coronary arteries once described diseased artery walls as looking as though they had been scrubbed by a brush, the result of multiple small injuries from the foods people have eaten and toxins that entered their bodies, leaving their marks over time. Every time the wall of the artery is injured—let's say after we eat a sticky bun at the mall—our bodies respond with inflammation. When inflammation persists, it ravages our blood vessels, and damaged blood vessels lead to heart disease.

Do you know what the deadliest disease on the planet earth is? Coronary artery disease. This occurs when those damaged, scratched-up arteries become narrow and unable to expand, making it difficult for blood to flow to the heart.

It is not caused by cholesterol in our diet. It is caused by constant assault from high blood pressure, sugar, refined carbohydrates, processed foods, excess body fat, and smoking—all of which precipitate chronic inflammation.

In recent years, coronary artery disease has killed about 7.4 million people in the world and 370,000 people in the United States annually. Here in the U.S., it's the leading cause of death for both women and men who are white, African American, and Hispanic. For Indigenous American, Alaska natives, and Asians or Pacific Islanders, heart disease is second only to cancer.

I'd be surprised if you didn't know someone who has had heart problems, but just in case, here's a list of a few famous people who suffered from heart attacks or heart disease: F. Scott Fitzgerald, Rosie O'Donnell, former president Bill Clinton, Barbara Walters, Toni Braxton, David Letterman, Larry King, Elizabeth Taylor, former vice president Dick Cheney, and Robin Williams.

We already know what causes atherosclerosis, but we'll review because, of course, these are the same things that cause heart problems: smoking, obesity, high blood pressure, diabetes, high blood sugar, stress, and lack of physical activity.

There is a clear link between diet and heart disease.

Former president Bill Clinton has publicly grappled with the question of how to best eat for his heart over the past ten years. Despite years of off-and-on dieting and exercising, by his last physical as president, he was 210 pounds. In 2004, at fifty-eight, he underwent an emergency quadruple-bypass operation. In February 2010, Clinton again suffered chest pain and was rushed in for emergency surgery. His doctors inserted two stents into one of his coronary arteries. Days after the surgery, Clinton started consulting with Dr. Dean Ornish, founder of the Preventive Medicine Research Institute and a major advocate for vegan diets. Based on the work and advice of Dr. Ornish, the author T. Colin Campbell (author of *The China Study*), and Caldwell Esselstyn, author of the 2007 book *Prevent and Reverse Heart Disease* and the star of the 2011 American documentary *Forks Over Knives*, Clinton became a vegan.

But based on the advice of Dr. Mark Hyman, the Clinton family's medical advisor and director of the Cleveland Clinic's Center for Functional Medicine, he began to add small amounts of salmon and eggs into his diet, opting for a Paleo-style diet with high-quality protein and natural fats, and low amounts of sugar and processed foods. Dr. Hyman, author of *The Blood Sugar Solution*, believes that sugar, not fat, causes heart disease. Studies have shown that high blood sugar causes insulin resistance, which creates inflammation in the endothelium and blood vessel injury that begins the process of atherosclerosis.

Ultimately, what Clinton realized, and what I want you to understand, is that what you eat and do with your body affects your blood flow, which affects your heart.

> ***TIPS:*** *Google and Verily (health subsidiary of Google) using artificial Intelligence (AI) have recently developed software to assess heart disease. By scanning the photos of blood vessels in the retina (behind the eye), AI algorithm can predict the future risk for heart attack and stroke—it has accuracy that is comparable to other more invasive tests. When you have a heart disease and need surgery or stent placement to bring more blood flow to the heart, know that the treatment is only temporary. Don't think that you now have brand-new blood vessels. Without lifestyle changes, coronary arteries will clog up again quickly. The changes must include adjusting your diet, weight and stress reduction, stopping smoking immediately, and increasing your physical activity.*

Stroke

A stroke, or "brain attack," happens when blood flow to an area in the brain is interrupted, depriving brain cells of oxygen and killing them. When brain cells die during a stroke, abilities controlled by that part of the brain—such as speech or muscle control—are lost. If you can visualize the brain as a computer, then a stroke is equivalent to wiping out the hard drive. It is difficult to recover and often devastating!

Every six seconds, somebody in the world dies of stroke—and in the United States, someone dies from a stroke every four minutes. About six million people die from strokes every year around the globe. And that number is rising. But a more shocking number is that fifteen million people suffer each year. Many are left with long-term disabilities like trouble speaking or understanding, paralysis or numbness in the face or arms or legs, and visual changes.

According to the World Health Organization, stroke is the second leading cause of death for people above the age of sixty, and the fifth leading cause of death in people fifteen to fifty-nine years old. One in six people worldwide will suffer a stroke in their lifetime. It is responsible for more deaths annually than AIDS, tuberculosis, and malaria combined. In the United States, stroke is the leading cause of adult disability.

So what is it, and what causes it?

There are two kinds of stroke—ischemic and hemorrhagic. A hemorrhagic stroke happens when a weakened or diseased vessel ruptures. The blood leaks into the surrounding brain. The accumulating blood compresses the brain and the pressure and swelling builds up. The blood flow to the brain slows and damage follows quickly.

The majority of strokes are ischemic in nature, which means that they occur as a result of blockage of blood flow to the brain. The underlying condition is usually atherosclerosis. It can cause two types of blockage that limit or cut off oxygen-rich blood to the brain. One is called *cerebral thrombosis*, which is a blood clot that develops at the narrowed part of the diseased blood vessel. But another type is *cerebral embolism*, when a blood clot or a piece of plaque is formed elsewhere (in the heart or in the arteries of upper chest or the neck) and travels up to the brain, blocking the blood vessel.

Sometimes there is a warning sign for a future stroke called *transient ischemic attack* (TIA). This occurs when there is a clot that forms usually due to a plaque. The most common symptom is loss of vision, but trouble speaking or weakness on one side of body is also seen. Luckily, TIA resolves within minutes, without any damage. However, the brain cells are especially sensitive to oxygen deprivation and permanent injury can occur from even a brief interruption in the blood flow.

Risk factors include anything that can cause chronic inflammation leading to blood vessel damage, which interferes with blood flow, including high blood pressure, diabetes, smoking, unhealthy diet, being overweight, stress and lack of physical activity.

TIP: Carotid Doppler Study (Ultrasound) is useful screening test for measuring the blood flow in your carotid artery (in the neck). As the artery narrows, there is a disturbance in the flow, which correlates with stroke risk.

Spot a stroke FAST.

Face drooping—Ask the person to smile. Is one side of the face droopy or numb?

Arm weakness—Ask the person to raise their arm. Is one side weak or drifts downward?

Speech difficulty—Speech is slurred or unable to speak. Ask the person to repeat a sentence.

Time to call 911—If the person shows any of these signs, call 911 and get them to the hospital ASAP.

Metabolic Syndrome

Do you have the proverbial spare tire or muffin top around your waist? That may be a sign of something more dangerous than simply not being able to button up your jeans. It may be a visible symptom encompassing a cluster of conditions called *metabolic syndrome*. These conditions individually and even more so collectively, lead to stiff blood vessels and inflammation.

Metabolic syndrome often starts with weight gain caused by inactivity and overindulgence on refined carbohydrates and processed foods, leading to higher blood sugar levels. One issue sets off another—the domino effect—and suddenly, the cells become insulin resistant, and insulin begins rising in the body, which leads to accelerated fat storage and an enlarged waistline. Hello, muffin top! As the lipid profile goes haywire and triglycerides rise, causing HDL to go down, you are put at even higher risk for cardiovascular

[84]

disease. As all of these problems converge, the damage to the blood vessels is overwhelming.

Most patients don't even know that they have metabolic syndrome, and most doctors aren't looking for it. In many cases, people are monitored for individual issues, not this syndrome. Many people who have it are not being treated for it. Postmenopausal women are at the highest risk for metabolic syndrome—about 33 to 42 percent of them have it already. Subtle in nature, one report showed that even a modest weight gain of five pounds over sixteen years could increase your chances of having metabolic syndrome by 45 percent. And if the circumference of your waist grows by four inches, your chances of suffering metabolic syndrome increase by 80 percent within five years.

As we age, our chances of developing metabolic syndrome increase exponentially because our body has much more difficulty processing sugar. The reasons: decreased metabolism, loss of muscle mass combined with simultaneous fat gain, a shift in hormone levels, and lower levels of physical activity. Blood sugar rises, weight gain follows, and eventually, a series of disease states begin, leading to metabolic syndrome. The number of people suffering from this syndrome is at epidemic levels in the United States.

It is an epidemic that has caused profound injury to the nation's blood vessels. Each disorder under the *metabolic* umbrella is dangerous when taken alone. But when combined, as the "deadly quartet"—which is high blood sugar, midsection obesity, high blood pressure, and a disturbance in lipid profile—metabolic syndrome has devastating inflammatory effects on the circulatory system. It is directly linked to heart attack and stroke.

Although metabolic syndrome is a hazardous condition, you can lessen your risks significantly by reducing your weight; increasing your physical activity; eating a diet low in sugar and rich in whole grains, fruits, vegetables, and fish; and working with your healthcare provider to monitor and manage blood glucose, blood lipid, and blood pressure. Lowering your blood sugar is the first step you must take in preventing or curing metabolic syndrome.

TIP: Don't let this syndrome sneak up on you. Be mindful that anyone can be susceptible. Start by reducing your refined carbs and sugar intake. Even moderate weight loss of

5 to10 percent can go a long way in reducing metabolic syndrome. Don't think you are safe because your waistline has not significantly increased.
A diabetic medication called metformin *can be started early to control your blood sugar (More on this in chapter 6.). Increasing physical activity with brisk walking, moving more, and/or aerobic exercise will help. As you age, be mindful of maintaining or increasing high levels of physical activity. Also, add grapefruit and cinnamon to your diet. Grapefruit helps with weight loss and cinnamon helps increase insulin sensitivity and decrease blood sugar.*

Alzheimer's Disease

One of the most feared diseases among the elderly is Alzheimer's disease (AD). It takes away your memory, and it places an enormous burden on families and doctors. Alzheimer's accounts for two-thirds of all causes of dementia and at this time there's no cure. It is thought that the accumulation of two proteins—amyloid plaques and tau tangles—cause progression of the disease. Although 244 drugs have been developed for AD since 2000, none have worked.

It is believed that Alzheimer's silently accelerates the atrophy of the hippocampus, a part of the brain that is critical for memory processing. Brain scans of people who have Alzheimer's exhibit hippocampi that are much more shrunken than people of the same age without the disease. And while it is known that those with APOE-e4 gene are at higher risk for developing Alzheimer's, the majority of those who acquire the disease do not possess this gene.

What is known is that circulation of blood through your brain can affect Alzheimer's. There is a close association between reduction of cerebral blood flow and the development of all neurodegenerative diseases (Alzheimer's, Parkinson's, Huntington's, Lou Gehrig's, and multiple sclerosis). There's no doubt that ample blood flow is essential to the health of the brain. In Alzheimer's, often there's an accompanying atherosclerotic blood vessel disease that impairs blood flow to the brain. In fact, patients who suffer strokes have a 60 percent increase in their risk for Alzheimer's. The diminished cerebral blood flow sets up a reduced clearance of amyloids, leading to plaque deposition in the brain.

[86]

Neuroinflammation also plays a central role in the pathogenesis of Alzheimer's disease. Chronic inflammation can be a deadly force inside the brain. More immune cells called *microglia* are found in the brains of AD patients. These inflammatory cells (microglia) are assigned with protecting the brain but can end up destroying normal neurons. Additionally, there's mounting evidence to indicate that microglia are participants in the propagation of plaques and tangles. As I've pointed out earlier, chronic inflammation means less blood flow and less oxygen, and that results in more brain cell damage or death.

A study out of Cleveland Clinic revealed that physically active volunteers with the APOE-e4 gene, meaning they were at higher risk for Alzheimer's disease, had brain scans that looked similar to the brain scans of people with much lower risk[9]. Exercise seemed to be protecting their brains! Meanwhile, the brains of volunteers who led sedentary lives appeared to be worsening. Other studies involving patients with mild cognitive impairment (risk for AD) who began an exercise regimen after six months showed improved brain scans and improved cognitive ability[10].

While researchers are unsure at this moment why exercise halts brain damage, they believe it involves the relationship between enhanced circulation and how the brain cleans up amyloid plaques and tau tangles. In addition, studies have shown that exercise improves the metabolism of fat and sugar in the brain while simultaneously calming inflammation.

TIP: *It is never too late to intervene when it comes to Alzheimer's or dementia. If you are at higher risk (positive for APOE-e4 gene, having had head injuries, have a family history of the disease, have suffered from heart disease, stroke, or diabetes; or have brain scan showing changes in the hippocampus), then it is important to take immediate steps to incorporate lifestyle changes to improve blood circulation to your brain. Exercise appears to be the most powerful tool in preventing Alzheimer's disease.*
Vegans and Vegetarians may become vitamin B$_{12}$ deficient, adding to the risk for AD. Be sure to check your levels.
Even if you are at low risk for AD, no one is immune from developing dementia. Increasing your physical activity and

modifying your diet to improve cardiovascular health is a better preventive tool than doing crossword puzzles to combat brain aging.

Cancer

Almost daily, we hear about a new vaccination or miracle drug to fight cancer by shrinking tumors or altering genes. President Nixon declared war on cancer in 1971, and despite incredible amounts of money, time, and genius being poured into cancer research and specifically the gene-mutation theory of cancer, that war is still being fought. The number of deaths from cancer has increased in the past twenty years. The sequencing of the human genome has propelled massive research into the genetic causes of cancer, and more than seven hundred high-tech drugs targeting unique DNA patterns of individual cancer cells have been developed—and not one of them has saved a single life. In fact, no single unifying genetic cause has been established in the race to cure cancer.

Cancer kills about 600,000 people a year in the United States, at the rate of about 1,600 cancer deaths every single day. In this year alone, there will be about 1.7 million new cancer cases. Within a few years, cancer will overtake heart disease as the leading killer of Americans, according to the American Cancer Society.

But why do we add cancer here, in our list of things in your body affected by circulation? Because convincing evidence is beginning to surface that oxygen delivery and blood nutrient content matters in the fight against cancer—both in terms of prevention and treatment.

First, what exactly is cancer? Besides being a metaphor for the worst things in life, it is a collection of about two hundred related diseases that all have this in common: some of the body's cells begin to divide uncontrollably and spread into surrounding tissue.

Cancer can happen anywhere in the human body, because the body is made of trillions of cells. Usually, normal cells grow and divide, so they can form new cells when your body needs them. When they get old or damaged, they die, with new cells replacing them.

When this organized system breaks down, that's cancer. Some cells become more and more irregular or abnormal, old and damaged cells don't die when they should, and new cells form when they aren't really necessary. All these extra cells start dividing without limit, and tumors start to form. Solid tumors are masses of tissue and are formed in many different kinds of cancer. Cancer in the blood, such as leukemia, does not form solid tumors.

If a tumor is deemed malignant, we call it cancer, which means it has the potential to spread into and invade surrounding tissues. Some cancer cells even break off and migrate by blood or the lymph system to far-off places in the body, forming new cancers that are distant from the original site; this is called *metastasis*.

Unique qualities allow cancer cells to grow out of control. They aren't specialized; they have no specific function other than to divide endlessly and live forever. They don't abide by the signals that usually tell cells to stop dividing or die, part of a process called *apoptosis*. They are able to get normal cells to feed them and form new blood vessels that supply them with nutrients and remove waste products. Cancer cells are no different from any other normal cells— they want to live, so they do this by building barriers around themselves to hide from the immune system, which removes damaged or abnormal cells.

The transition from a normal cell to a malignant cancer has long been believed to be driven by changes to a cell's DNA, which is housed in a cell's nucleus. That's the conventional theory—that cancer typically originates during a person's lifetime because of a series of genetic injuries or copying mistakes inside the nucleus. These mutations lead, eventually, from a passive, normal cell to a deadly, aggressively regenerative cell, or so the theory goes. But researchers haven't found the mutation that causes cancer. They've found between 1,000 and 10,000 mutations (in the DNA) in most adult cancers, and in some cancers, like lung cancer and melanoma, there have been more than 100,000 different mutations identified. Would it even be possible to come up with a treatment that targets that many mutations? Or maybe something else is happening, something that triggered those mutations that could be prevented.

What if cancer doesn't start with mutations in our DNA? Scientists universally agree that cellular changes causing cancer begin with exposure to carcinogens like radiation, toxins, ultraviolet rays, virus, tobacco smoke, and asbestos. The damage from these carcinogens may result in direct injury to the DNA. But they can also lead to inflammation and disruption of architectural integrity of blood vessels, causing slowed blood flow and low oxygen delivery to cells.

Enter Otto Warburg, a German physiologist and Nobel laureate who, in 1934, published his treatise titled "The Prime Cause and Prevention of Cancer." Warburg's research showed that cancer cells were low in oxygen, and the normal process of respiration was replaced by fermentation—a less-efficient process that converts sugar to energy without using oxygen or mitochondria. "All normal cells have an absolute requirement for oxygen, but cancer cells can live without oxygen—a rule without exception," he said. "Deprive a cell of 35 percent of its oxygen for forty-eight hours, and it may become cancerous." He believed that defective mitochondria were responsible for cancer genesis.

Currently, mutations of DNA contained in the nucleus are thought to cause cancer among most of the scientific community. However, there is a growing body of evidence suggesting that issues outside of the nucleus are involved in the formation of cancer. Recent research has attributed mitochondria to cancer-gene suppression and their dysfunction play a pivotal role in the development and progression of cancer. Mitochondria are also involved in cell death (apoptosis). Apoptosis is lost in cancer cells, as they continue to live and divide forever. Mitochondria are the power plants in our cells that consume 80 to 90 percent of the oxygen during respiration. Normal cells use respiration to efficiently turn any kind of nutrient (fat, carbohydrate, or protein) into high amounts of energy. This process requires oxygen and breaks food down completely into harmless carbon dioxide and water. In contrast, many cancer cells do not use oxygen to produce energy even when it is available (Warburg effect). These findings have led to the rebirth of the metabolic theory of cancer first proposed by Warburg, in which altered energy metabolism rather than genetic mutations is the main driver in cancer.

What if I told you that certain cells choose to become cancer? Maybe malignant transformation is an evolutionary process (both Darwinian and Lamarckian) adopted by our cells. And cancer is a mechanism utilized by our cells to survive hypoxia (a low oxygen state). So here's another plausible way that our circulation can play a profound role in cancer: Inflammation and injury choke off the blood flow to cells and tissues, creating hypoxia. Since oxygen dictates the microenvironment of cells, and hypoxia is the most pertinent physiological stressor (when oxygen level falls, cells produce considerably less energy and accumulate substantially more toxic metabolic waste), the entire cell is now in jeopardy. Eventually, prolonged hypoxia exerts selection pressure on these cells to evolve and live with less oxygen. Because our cells possess plasticity—the ability of cells to change their identity—reprogramming of DNA (via DNA mutations or alterations in expression) can occur and allow them to live on as cancer cells. Cancerous changes may actually be an adaptive response by our cells to avoid dying from harsh conditions like hypoxia—born in a low oxygen environment, cancer cells have a competitive advantage and can thrive in this setting.

If hypoxia leads to cancer, then sugar feeds it. Growing cancer requires more and more sugar. Where does that sugar come from? Your diet.

A study of mice injected with aggressive breast cancer shows that sugar is essential for cancer growth. Mice were placed into three groups of twenty-four, according to their blood sugar levels[11]. After seventy days, sixteen of the mice with high blood sugar levels had died, eight mice with normal blood sugar had died, and only one of the mice with low blood sugar had died. The mice with the lowest blood sugar levels were much better at surviving cancer.

Also, there's an imaging test called a *positron emission tomography (PET) scan* that is used for cancer detection that depends upon cancer's quest for sugar. In the PET scan, a patient's blood vessels are infused with radioactive sugar. Since cancers are highly metabolic and consume sugar much faster than the normal cells, the radioactive sugar will light up the area(s) that contain cancer cells. The faster growing the cancer, the more sensitive the PET scan—more evidence that cancer loves sugar.

This doesn't necessarily mean eating sugar or sugary food will cause cancer. But a diet containing high amounts of sugar will eventually lead to elevation of blood sugar. It's evident in human studies that elevated blood sugar is clearly linked to cancer.

Researchers have known of an association between diabetes and cancer since 1932, but why elevated blood sugar would increase the risk of cancer is still unclear. We know that high blood sugar promotes free radical formation and chronic inflammation, and

[91]

makes blood sticky, slowing blood flow and ultimately reducing oxygen delivery to the cells. Insulin resistance and elevated blood insulin levels are proinflammatory, and have additional independent risk factors for cancer. Since cancer cells begin with injury and inflammation and have high affinity for sugar, it's logical that a drug that lowers blood sugar would help fight cancer. As it turns out, a medication that is already being used to combat diabetes called *metformin* is precisely that. Metformin lowers blood sugar and blood insulin level. A number of studies on diabetics have shown metformin use results in reduction in cancer rates when compared with other diabetic medications. New evidence is showing benefits of metformin in lowering cancer rates among nondiabetic patients.

Another up-and-coming area of study in the war on cancer is exercise—or increasing the flow rate of oxygen-carrying blood to the tissues. At the Lee Jones Lab in the Memorial Sloan Kettering Cancer Research Institute in New York City, researchers are studying how exercise can be used before, during, and after cancer treatment to enhance chemotherapy response. They are also looking at whether exercise itself could be an effective treatment for cancer.

Here's one way exercise has already proven useful: Many cancers are resistant to treatment because they have generated chaotic and entwined web of dysfunctional blood vessels that oxygen levels surrounding the cancer are very low. Cancers can flourish in a hypoxic (low-oxygen) environment. Since chemotherapy drugs and radiation target cells with normal blood flow, the cancers are often protected from the toxic effects of chemotherapy and radiation. By exercising, the blood flow will increase, bringing more oxygen and stabilizing the cancer site—making treatments much more effective.

In a paper published in March 2015 in the *Journal of the National Cancer Institute*, researchers at the Duke Cancer Institute found that, in mice induced with tumors, exercise led to both improved function and increased number of blood vessels around the tumors, enhancing oxygen flow to the cancer site. What was surprising in their study was that the tumor growth slowed substantially in mice with exercise alone, and when exercise was combined with chemotherapy, the tumor growth slowed even more, especially compared to the rapid tumor growth seen in the inactive group.

Exercise is beneficial for patients recuperating from cancer treatment, and it helps lower the chance of recurrence. It improves the structure of blood vessels, stimulates blood vessels to enlarge, increases the red blood cell count, and creates many new capillaries, bringing more blood flow and oxygen to cells. It also contributes to healthier lipid profile and lowering blood sugar level.

TIPS: Cancer patients and survivors should try to get the same amount of exercise recommended for the general population, about 150 minutes a week of moderate-intensity aerobic exercise. Resistance training and stretching also are recommended. Among other benefits, regular exercise will improve the mood and strengthen the immune system, resulting in better tolerance and response to cancer treatments.

Hyperbaric Oxygen Therapy (HBOT) is used as an adjunctive treatment for many conditions, especially when there's low oxygen in the tissues, such as diabetes, smoking, or compromised blood flow. HBOT is the delivery of oxygen at higher-than-normal atmospheric pressure. Patients are put in a pressure chamber with 100 percent oxygen. Since many cancers contain areas that are poorly oxygenated, HBOT can overcome oxygen deficient regions. It can also aid in chemo and radiation therapy and make treatments more effective. It compensates for damaged blood vessels by forcing more oxygen throughout the body and supports tissues that are hypoxic. However, HBOT is not for everyday use. It can cause toxicity to normal cells.

Ask your doctor about a ketogenic diet as an aid in the battle against cancer. Cancer consumes large amounts of sugar to generate enough energy; a diet low in carbohydrates, high in fats, and high-quality protein helps the body burn ketone bodies as energy and deprive cancer cells of sugar.

I also recommend taking metformin as an adjuvant therapy for cancer. Metformin will keep your sugar level lower and improve your insulin function (more in chapter 6).

Chapter 5: Linking Aging to Our Circulation

The key to aging well and living healthy longer is a well-cared-for circulatory system. A consistent, reliable blood flow that can nourish cells over the years is the true fountain of youth. The result of diseased blood vessels is a whole litany of familiar problems that can be summed up under one heading: aging.

The Aging Process

Aging is one of the most complex biological processes, and its mechanism is still being hotly pursued in laboratories and debated among scientists around the world. Let's get this straight—*aging is not a disease and it is absolutely going to happen to every one of us*. It's a part of the experience of being alive, and it's inevitable. You're born, you die, and everything in between is aging. It's part of being human. But can it be delayed? Can you live healthier longer? And how does the circulatory system factor into that equation?

In the past one hundred years, public health measures have been made to combat infectious diseases, improve the quality of our water, and prepare and store our food with an eye toward sanitary precautions. Lives have been saved for sure. But aging itself—the process of aging—has not been slowed at all during that time. Researchers haven't come close to figuring it out. And the truth is that the more reputable researchers are not looking for age extension as much as they are looking for an extension of the period of healthy life people live (healthspan). People might live a little longer, but the true goal is to live healthier. I believe that keeping your circulatory system clean—staving off blood vessel damage and maintaining brisk blood flow—is your best chance.

Researchers in the past decade have come to agree on the "pillars of aging" that affect cell metabolism, cell growth, response to stress, stem cell vigor, inflammation and protein maintenance, and quality control within cells. We know that aging occurs in all living things. We grow from infants to toddlers to youth and preteens and go through puberty and ultimately transition into adults and then continue to progress through different stages of adulthood, which generally include gray hair and menopause—and we're positive that aging occurs at a very cellular level. But what does that mean exactly? Your body is made up of thirty-seven trillion (that's right, *trillion*) cells. Each organ and each body part is made up of tissues, and each tissue is designed with billions of cells, most of them pretty similar.

As cells age, they also get bigger, less able to divide and multiply, pigmented, and filled with fatty substances. They don't function as well as they used to, and the organs they make up start to malfunction too. Cells are born with an expiration date—they cannot live forever.

But what causes cells to age? Genetics? Environmental damage?

Extreme heat and radiation virtually cook a cell and result in cell death. But toxins from pollution, smoke, and food can also harm cells—the same things that cause atherosclerosis (our blood vessels are the first to be exposed and continue to be affected by circulating toxins). Cells can be injured directly, but they can also suffocate to death from damaged blood vessels that can't deliver enough oxygen to them.

In terms of genes, it's true that you were born with a set of genes inherited from your parents and those same genes will stay with you for your entire life. While some of them can become defective and can contribute to disease in your body, most are perfectly capable of carrying people to a very old age. And how much significance do genes play anyway? Studies have shown that they account for about 25 to 30 percent of the aging process. The rest? Totally up to you and how you optimize your healthspan. That's the only way currently known to increase your lifespan— *lifestyle choices impact your health and your length and quality of life*.

A young, healthy body is like a new car with very few miles on it. Reckless lifestyle choices don't impact your body immediately, which is probably why more people make them. However, as we age, these choices slowly accumulate, and our bodies begin to show symptoms.

The biology of aging is a complicated mystery, but scientists have come to agree that aging either is on a biologic timetable similar to the one that regulates childhood growth and development, or that it is caused by damage inside the body from various environmental factors.

[95]

Most scientists agree that too many free radicals accelerate aging. Free radicals are molecules that contain an unpaired electron, which make them unstable and destructive forces inside blood vessels. They are often the origin of a chain reaction, which damages molecules and cells, sometimes causing them to die. Free radicals can occur because of exposure to cigarette smoke, air pollutants, high blood sugar, fried foods, alcohol, industrial chemicals, stress, and even excessive exercise, but they can also arise as a byproduct of basic cell metabolism. The damage they inflict can be directly linked to inflammation, atherosclerosis, heart disease, cancer, and early aging.

TIP: Neutralize free radicals with antioxidants found especially in fruits and vegetables, but that are also produced by our bodies at times, such as during moderate exercise. Antioxidants are special molecules that can safely interact with free radicals and terminate the chain reaction before damage occurs.

Chronological Versus Biological Age

When asked your age, you may be quick to give a number based on how many years you've been alive since you were born. That's your chronological age. But chronological age may or may not reflect how you feel, look, and perform, nor is it a good predictor of how much longer you might have to live. That's up to you. And that's reflected in your biological age. This can be measured objectively, and it can give you a good idea of how your lifestyle may be speeding up your aging process. Biological age refers to the "real" age of the person's body based on various biomarkers. Biomarkers are measurable indicators of the severity of or presence of some disease state or what condition your body is in and how it is functioning. Recent studies confirmed that biological age was much more accurate than chronological age in predicting mortality[12]. There are five biomarkers of aging—physical and cognitive capability, physiological, endocrine and immune functions.

Picture a car that has fifty thousand miles on it but looks and drives like new. You're not surprised to find the owner pampered and cared for the car—regular oil changes, high-grade gasoline, tune-ups, immediate response to warning lights, and safe driving that didn't stress the engine. The car was kept in the garage and away

[96]

from harsh element. So how have you taken care of your body—specifically, your circulatory system? If you've treated your body, and especially your circulatory system, right, while the calendar tells you you're fifty-one, you may actually be only thirty-five inside.

Once you see how you measure up, you can reverse your biological age dramatically by changing your lifestyle to get your blood pumping and moving. Remember—blood feeds oxygen and nutrients to every cell in your body. Maybe you're fifty but you test sixty-four. Or maybe you're sixty but testing like a forty-year-old.

There are certain things we've come to expect with each decade—societal norms assigned to chronological age—and we trace them here up to a hundred years, which currently only about one person in ten thousand lives beyond.

First decade (age 0 to 9)—age of dependency. We're fed and cleaned, learn to walk and talk, and eventually start our education. You grow baby teeth, lose them, and replace them with adult teeth.

Second decade (age 10 to 19)—discovery of sexuality. Suddenly, our hormones rage and we are aware of the opposite sex. We go through puberty somewhere around the age of thirteen. During these years, teens also lose their ability to hear high-frequency sounds, learn to act less impulsively, live within the rules of society, and develop the ability to think logically.

Third decade (age 20 to 29)—early adulthood. We feel independent. We try to find a comfortable niche within society with our first real job and our own partner and family. The cognitive process starts a slow decline in the midtwenties; our body has assumed its adult shape; we have finished formal education and accumulated intellectual knowledge. Many feel these years are the peak of their lives as the majority are healthy and have fewer responsibilities.

Fourth decade (age 30 to 39)—the prime of life. We have figured out how the world works. We think that we know what we want, and we raise our children, plan our future, usually enjoy more financial security and good health, and do not worry about disease.

Fifth decade (age 40 to 49)—middle age. We don't exactly feel old during this decade but are aware of the fact that the chances of living to twice this age are not very good. We may have a midlife crisis that forces us to evaluate our life and try to make changes, but it is not easy because we have to live within the constraints of our work, family structure, and social environment. There's an abrupt change in our physical shape, our vision begins to deteriorate, and we become more forgetful. Some of us experience considerable hair loss and/or graying hair. Slightly weak and vulnerable now, for the first time, activities that used to seem easy become tougher for us, but not for our children, who seem to have overtaken us. Your career might be at its peak, and your earning potential the highest it will ever be, but you're still aware of the aging happening.

Sixth decade (age 50 to 59)—age of biological decline. We become aware of wrinkles, gray hair, arthritis pains, menopause, and decreased libido. Having entered the back nine of your life, you're suddenly eligible for membership in AARP, you need reading glasses, and your body becomes pear shaped.

Seventh decade (age 60 to 69)—retirement age. You become eligible for Medicare. If you are lucky and have planned well, you can stop working and start traveling or doing community service. Maybe you take medicine for diabetes, high cholesterol, blood thinning, or high blood pressure. Your joints begin to hurt, and you may be less energetic, although you may be expecting or already have some grandchildren. Napping may become a welcome regular daily event, and work may no longer be the most important thing on your mind. Instead of vigorous workouts, you take nice walks.

Eighth decade (age 70 to 79)—age of decreased mobility. Now a full-fledged senior citizen, the little pains of twenty years ago have increased and now restrict normal activities. You may walk with a hunch because osteoporosis has begun. Facial wrinkles become much more pronounced. Maybe you use a cane, have had hernia or cataract surgery, and your age spots are hard to cover. You move slower and you become shorter. Your circle of friends starts to shrink as heart attacks, strokes, and cancer take their toll. Maybe your children are your guardians, or you are in a nursing home because you can no longer take care of yourself. Mortality and life reflection preoccupy your mind.

Ninth decade (age 80 to 89)—age of assisted living. Even if we can still take care of ourselves, we may need somebody to help us clean the house, go shopping for us, or prepare our food. Health problems become more severe. We may become incontinent and have to wear adult diapers. Most people will not live beyond this decade. You may have lost your spouse.

Tenth decade (age 90 to 99)—pre-centenarian.
Congratulations! If you've made it this far, you are one of the lucky ones. What did you do right to be here? Good genes? Fewer severe health problems? Good family support? If you are still active, you may live to be a centenarian. The life expectancy at age ninety is 3.8 years, and by age ninety-nine the life expectancy drops to 2.1 years. Every day may be a struggle for life. There can be digestive problems, cardiovascular problems, mobility problems, or immune system problems on any given day.

So, again, how old are you? And would you like to be younger, biologically speaking? Even if you scored the same as your chronological age, you can do better! Wouldn't you love to say, "I was born in 1965, but I am actually twenty-seven years old"?

Let us know how you measured up. Is your biological age older than your chronological age? Don't worry. If you start now, by changing your nutrition and exercise patterns and getting rid of bad habits, you can reverse the trajectory. Stop wrecking your circulatory system—that's where the bad news begins. If you are younger than your chronological age, congratulations! Now let's do better. And don't settle for average, because the average Joe American…well, he's not that healthy.

TIPS: *Here are some simple exercises, courtesy of health educator, consultant to Olympians, and biochemist Stephen Cherniske, you might do at home to check your biological age[13].*
Skin elasticity: Lay your hand down on a desk or table, palm down. Pinch the skin at the back of your hand for five seconds. Let go and time how long it takes your skin to go back to its smooth appearance. If you're very young, it should snap back immediately. An average forty-five-year-old's skin will take three to five seconds. At age sixty, it takes about ten to fifteen seconds on average. By the time you are seventy, it usually takes thirty-five to sixty seconds to crawl back. So, if you are sixty and it takes three to five seconds, this test indicates your biological age is around forty-five.
Reaction time: Ask someone to hold an eighteen-inch ruler or yardstick vertically from the one-inch line. Place your thumb and index finger about three inches apart at the eighteen-

inch line. Ask your partner to let go without warning you. Then catch the ruler as fast as you can between your thumb and index finger. Mark down the number on the ruler where you catch it. Do this three times and average your score. A twenty-year-old will average about twelve inches. That generally decreases progressively to about five inches by the time you are sixty-five or about 1.75 inches per decade. So if your score is 7.5 inches, you test out at about age fifty for reaction time. Games like Ping-Pong, tennis, and foosball can have positive impact on your scores.

<u>Static balance:</u> Take off your shoes and stand on a level uncarpeted surface with your feet together. Close your eyes and raise your right foot about six inches off the ground if you are right-handed, or on your left foot if you are left-handed. See how many seconds you can stand that way without opening your eyes or moving your supporting foot. Most twenty-year-olds can do it easily for thirty seconds or more. By age sixty-five, most people can only stand for three to five seconds. You lose about six seconds a decade, so if you score twelve to fourteen seconds, you test at about fifty years of age. Yoga, balance board training, and exercise can improve your scores.

<u>Vital lung capacity:</u> Take three deep breaths and hold the fourth without forcing it. Healthy twenty-year-olds can hold it for two minutes easily. We lose about 15 percent, or eighteen seconds per decade, so a sixty-year-old will do well to hold it for forty-five seconds. If you can hold your breath for sixty-five seconds, you test at about the fifty-year-old level. You can improve with exercise and deep breathing techniques.

<u>Memory/cognition:</u> Ask a friend to write down three random seven-digit numbers without showing them to you. Ask him or her to say the first string of seven numbers twice. Now repeat the string backward. Do the same for the other two numbers and average the results. A thirty-year-old should score 100 percent. Most of the fifty-year-olds will miss one digit out of seven. Most of the sixty-year-olds will miss two, and seventy-year-olds will miss three.

[100]

Premature Aging

So, we've talked about biological aging, but what about premature aging? Are we aging too fast? Is that decade list earlier correct, or are the norms we look for per decade actually signs that people are aging prematurely?

There's a fascinating cohort study out of Dunedin, New Zealand, that weighed in on premature aging in 2015. It's called, appropriately, the Dunedin Multidisciplinary Health and Development Study and it's an ongoing longitudinal study of the health, development, and well-being of 1,037 people who were born between 1972 and 1973 in Dunedin, New Zealand. Researchers have gathered information from three generations of the same family relating to cardiovascular, respiratory, oral, sexual, reproductive, mental health; lifestyle risk factors; and psychosocial functioning. Since age three, the people in the study have been assessed every two years up to age fifteen and then at age eighteen, twenty-one, twenty-six, thirty-two, and thirty-eight. The study members will be seen again at forty-four and forty-five. During an assessment, they are brought back to Dunedin (two-thirds live outside of New Zealand) for an intensive day of interviews, physical exams, blood tests, and questionnaires.

At the age thirty-eight assessment, 96 percent of all living eligible study members, or 961 people, participated. Recent findings from the study, published in July 2015, explain why the people at their twenty-year high school reunion (who would all be about thirty-eight) appear to be aging at such different rates.

First of all, they actually *are* aging at very different rates. The function of their kidneys, liver, lungs, and metabolic and immune systems are all aging, and the changes in these organs and systems shows up in eyes, joints, hair, and teeth. Although most of the participants did not have chronic disease, their biological age varied greatly from twenty-eight to sixty-one.

Measuring for pace of aging, researchers found most of them aged about one year biologically for every chronological year. But some were aging as fast as three years per one chronological year. And some of them were aging zero years for each chronological year.

The conclusion was that aging doesn't only happen late in life. Signs of aging are apparent at twenty-six and more so at thirty-

[101]

eight. Study members who were aging faster scored lower on tests of balance and coordination, walking upstairs, and solving unfamiliar problems. When Duke University students were asked to look at pictures of the study participants and guess their ages, the students always guessed a higher age for the participants whose biological age was higher. Not only were their bodies acting older and their biological functions older, but they also looked older. Only 20 percent of that is attributable to genes, say the researchers, noting environmental factors play a huge role.

So, here's what we extract from all that: As a society, we've accepted a standard of aging based on how our average population ages. Some age faster, some age what we consider to be appropriately, and some don't seem to age much at all. Listen, we know that we will all age regardless of our genes or how carefully we live. We are going to age. But maybe we are aging too fast. Most people possess biological age that exceeds their chronological years. Perhaps it's the people in the Dunedin study that didn't appear to age much—less than a year per chronological year—who are the ones that are aging normally. Maybe they should be the standard. Maybe thirty-eight doesn't look like thirty-eight but looks *younger* than what we associate with thirty-eight right now. Guessing someone's age is always relative to what we think the norm is. Maybe the norm for any age should look better and younger than it does right now if people were to take care of their bodies, especially their circulatory systems.

> *TIPS: While plastic surgery can help fight the external appearance of premature aging, my best medical advice to truly turn back the internal biological clock is to start following your biomarkers. Recently proposed biomarkers for healthy aging include measuring blood pressure, fasting blood sugar, hemoglobin A1c, bone mineral density, and blood lipids. Each of these tests for biomarkers is disease defining, while they are also all linked to the health of your blood vessels. And the very best way to improve your biomarkers is to modify your lifestyle.*

Blue Zone

Back in 2004, the *National Geographic* explorer and educator Dan Buettner teamed up with the world's best longevity

[102]

experts to research areas around the globe where people reach the age of one hundred ten times more often than in the United States.

Mr. Buettner likes to call these places where people forgot to die "blue zones." Dan and *National Geographic* took teams of scientists to five locations to identify lifestyle characteristics that might explain that longevity. The locales they visited were Ikaria, Greece; Okinawa, Japan; Sardinia, Italy; the Nicoya peninsula in Costa Rica; and a community of Seventh-Day Adventists in Loma Linda, California.

They were able to identify behavioral and lifestyle characteristics that all these communities shared—and to which they attributed the high rates of longevity and fewer instances of dementia and other chronic illnesses often associated with aging. In all five communities, people engage in physical activity regularly, take in a moderate level of calories, have strong family and community connections, experience low levels of stress, and believe that they have a sense of purpose. All these factors together culminate in societies that have clean circulatory systems.

Nutritionally, they eat whole-food, plant-based diets that feature fruits, vegetables, whole grains, and small amounts of meat. Beans are a popular protein. And nobody relies on supplements or pills to keep them healthy.

Being physical is part of their daily lives—they walk everywhere, do their own chores, and aren't spending time weightlifting or in organized exercise classes. It is significant to note that in all communities, elderly people are valued and families gather around them as they age and treat them like important, significant people.

This contrasts sharply with the American concept of aging, which often involves deterioration of health, dependency on others, and a dysfunctional social system. Many people regard old age with fear about disabilities, being a burden on loved ones, and the inevitability of nursing home living. Protecting and supporting our circulatory system can ease some of those concerns and possibly lead to lives like citizens of the blue zones. In Sardinia, a 104-year-old man can still chop wood for the midday fire. A 103-year-old Okinawan woman grows her own vegetables, tends them, and gathers them for meals. In Ikaria, a ninety-year-old man tends his sheep. Growing old with a healthy body and an active mind is the return on the investment of a life filled with activity and healthy food choices.

> *TIPS: Movement doesn't have to be done at the gym. Be active by mowing the grass, walking to town, taking the stairs instead of elevators, and participating in activities as much as you can. Don't think getting old means you should sit down and stop moving. Eat a plant-based diet with less meat and limited processed food. Drinking wine with this type of diet will increase the absorption of flavonoids (berries, citrus fruits, cocoa) by three times as compared to drinking wine with a steak. Studies have shown that people who feel like they are part of a community live up to eight years longer. So you should stay engaged no matter what your chronological age shows—stay relevant and always have a sense of purpose.*

Research on Aging

In the summer of 2015, Ancestry DNA, a leader in consumer genetics, and Calico, a longevity research arm of Google, partnered to investigate the genetics of human lifespan. Between them, they have access to the anonymous genetic database from millions of people. Their findings recently published in *Genetics* revealed that heritability of longevity was less than 10 percent, much lower than the previous estimates, according to these researchers.

Searching for longevity genes is the new frontier, with many wealthy entrepreneurs, researchers, and governments looking for the fountain of youth. For instance, the Palo Alto Longevity Prize is offering $1 million to research teams who can create and explain dramatic increases in lifespans and health of lab rats and mice.

Already studies comparing the lifespans of identical twins compared to fraternal show that longevity is influenced about 25 percent by genes and 75 percent by other factors, including lifestyle choices. But the specific genes that contribute to longevity have been elusive.

Researchers at Stanford University and other centers have sequenced the genes of seventeen centenarians in good health in search of genetic clues to how they've managed to live so well for so long. One of them practiced as a physician in Georgia until she was 103 and another was a stockbroker on Wall Street until the age of

109, both still in good physical and mental health. In fact, all the participants maintained high levels of cognitive and physical function throughout their entire lives. Although one individual had Alzheimer's disease and another had survived cancer, centenarians were able to escape many age-related diseases. In a separate study, centenarians exhibited elevated levels of HDL, which could explain their longevity.

Thus far, they haven't found any gene variants that stand out. One gene, called TSHZ3, was slightly enriched in the centenarians, but the levels were not higher than usual. They did find one of the long-living individuals carried a potentially pathogenic gene for the breast and ovarian cancer (BRCA1 gene), and another supercentenarian (someone living beyond 110) carried a gene mutation that's been linked to a heart condition. That supercentenarian actually lived to be the world's oldest man.

No known human being in the history of the world has ever lived past 130 years. It's highly unlikely you have a shot at making it past 110, to be honest, although a noted researcher on aging, Steven N. Austad, has bet fellow researchers one million dollars that at least one 150-year-old person will be alive in 2050.

At the present time, in the United States, older ages are considered between seventy-five and ninety, and most people die somewhere in between those years due to the biological mechanisms of aging. At this moment, nobody has figured out how to change those processes. The more relevant question than that of life expectancy is health span—how healthy are the years that you live? While people are living longer due to treatments for cancer and other chronic diseases—there will be 524 million people over sixty-five years across the globe by 2050—there will also be 83.7 million disabled elderly people in the United States by that year too.

Governments, universities, and private organizations are busy trying to unlock the secrets of the biological aging process. There are several ongoing studies that consider what it means to get older and why certain people seem to have an easier time of it than others.

The National Institute on Aging's Baltimore Longitudinal Study of Aging (BLSA), which began in 1958, is the longest-running scientific study of human aging. Much of our current knowledge of aging comes from the study, especially the facts that natural aging doesn't cause diabetes, hypertension, or dementia and that there is no accurate chronological timetable for human aging. Everybody ages differently!

One project within the Baltimore study is Insight into Determinants of Exceptional Aging and Longevity (IDEAL), which looks at "exceptional agers," people eighty or older who are healthy and have no physical or cognitive limitations. What clues can these volunteers offer about how to age better?

Up in Canada, researchers have taken on an even more ambitious twenty-year study with fifty thousand participants between the ages of forty-five and eighty. By looking at the biological, medical, psychological, social, and economic aspects of their lives, researchers on the Canadian Longitudinal Study on Aging (CLSA) hope to look at how all these factors combined shape the way people age.

In Okinawa, Japan, a study of centenarians has been going on since 1975 in hopes of revealing the genetic and lifestyle factors accounting for their longevity. You see, the folks in Okinawa live the longest and the healthiest in the world. Like many people who live over one hundred, diseases come late in life and they age slowly, often escaping dementia, heart disease, stroke, and cancer. It's been thought that genetics is involved in about one-third of the nine hundred plus centenarians studied.

The idea that our lifestyle plays a much bigger role than our genes in determining longevity is universally accepted. An emerging concept called *epigenetics,* which looks at how the environment modifies the behavior of our genes, has been a paradigm shift in the way we think about the DNA. Numerous studies investigating the influence of epigenetics on the DNA to lengthen lifespan is the hot topic today.

> **TIPS:** *While research is ongoing and likely many years away from benefitting the average person regarding having their genes meddled with, know that lifestyle changes can have a profound and beneficial impact on your genes through epigenetic changes. There are some practical things that you can do today to give yourself a better shot at surviving longer. Learn from people who eat healthy, then teach your family and friends to eat better and surround yourself with friends who are also interested in fitness and walk a*

[106]

lot. Being self-disciplined, organized, and focused is also a trait of people who live longer. So is foregoing a housekeeper and doing your own mopping and cleaning. Spending time with family, nurturing spirituality, and having a purpose in life ranked high in the lifestyles of people from both Okinawa and Sardinia, which have the highest numbers of centenarians in the world.

Aging Blood Vessels

Canadian physician Sir William Osler, one of the four founding professors of Johns Hopkins Hospital and considered the father of modern medicine, was often quoted as saying, "We are as old as our arteries."

. We now know that the heart has a natural pacemaker (or the sinus node that generates an electrical impulse). As we age, some of the pathways of this system may develop scars and fat deposits, and the natural pacemaker loses some of its cells. These changes may result in a slightly slower heart rate. Also, our older hearts may be a little bigger than our younger hearts, with thicker walls, which means chambers hold less blood and the heart fills with blood more slowly. It's also normal for the heart to have aging pigment, for the muscles to degenerate a little bit, and for the valves to thicken, become stiffer, and cause a heart murmur.

Age also means reduced sensitivity in the receptors that monitor our blood pressure. The walls of our arteries thicken and stiffen, which cause elevation in the pressure when the heart beats. In our capillaries, walls thicken too, while their numbers decrease, which reduces nutrient and gas exchange. Our ability to make new blood vessels falls. There's an overall drop in blood volume accompanied by drop in hemoglobin, which carries oxygen to our tissues. Nitric oxide—vital for the vessels ability to expand—is less plentiful. Our flexible, elastic vessels become more like rusty, rigid pipes. Plaque buildup in our arteries is a progressive process that continues with age.

Is that inevitable? Is it preventable? Should we just shrug our shoulders and accept it as part of the aging process? Nope.

No matter what your age, even three months of brisk walking can change the flexibility of your blood vessels. Studies show that older athletes have blood vessels that function the same as younger people's. Long-term exercise protects our circulatory system from constant damage we subject it to our entire lives.

New research on aging blood vessels has taken scientists to revive an old idea called *parabiosis*—surgically joining the circulatory systems. In the lab, when old mice skin was sewed to younger mice (much like a Siamese twin), all the tissues and the organs of the older mice began to rejuvenate, making the older mice stronger, smarter, healthier, and even their fur shinier. Shared circulation revitalized the blood flow of the older mice resulting in fountain of youth effect.

A robust blood flow is what keeps us healthy—it's also the breakdown that eventually fails us. Dying of natural causes means that our heart stops pumping, blood stops moving, and our circulatory system comes to an end (called *circulatory arrest*). If it ceases to deliver life-sustaining substances (oxygen and nutrients), then our cells will age quickly and die. Blood vessels are the true lifeline for our cells. It is never too late to meet the challenge of the wise Dr. Osler, who knew that our age isn't the number of our years but the health of our blood vessel.

Blood Vessel Wall
Blood flow is profoundly shaped by the surrounding blood vessel wall. The wall is composed of three different layers and the blood pressure determines its thickness (higher pressure means a thicker wall), and these cells need oxygen and nutrients too. Oxygen diffuses directly from the bloodstream through the inner wall (endothelium), but as the wall gets thicker (as in medium to large arteries), it needs a secondary source of oxygen that is provided by the vasa vasorum. The vasa vasorum is an intricate network of tiny vascular highways that penetrate the walls of the blood vessels from outside to deliver oxygen and nutrients to the outer and middle part of the artery. Vascular smooth muscle (remember this muscle is responsible for the flexibility of blood vessels), which makes up the majority of the wall, resides predominantly in the

middle layer and is most vulnerable to hypoxic injury.

Damage to the endothelium or problem in the vasa vasorum will block oxygen delivery to the blood vessel wall (both resulting from injury and chronic inflammation). As oxygen supply dwindles, smooth muscle cells kick in their adaptive response—they survive *hypoxia* by multiplying and morphing— behaving much like cancer. Smooth muscle cells are re-programmed and altered, becoming a major player in atherosclerosis and even laying down calcium deposits (resembling a bone) within the blood vessel wall, thereby hardening the artery. Not only does the wall thicken and stiffen, but it also becomes brittle. When the blood vessel wall is further oxygen deprived, it's more prone to rupture. Recent studies have shown that vascular smooth muscle is intimately involved in all aspects of plaque formation. With blood vessel wall injury— the healing process is orchestrated by the repair apparatus of the smooth muscle'—plaque is the end result.

Restore Circulation and Live Longer and Healthier

So how old are you? Is it determined by the number of your years or the condition of your body? Can you preserve your life, perhaps live a little longer and healthier? Earlier, it was covered that at the root of chronic disease, cancer, atherosclerosis, and premature aging, you'll find a common thread involving injury and inflammation of the blood vessels. Is this a coincidence or a continuum of this same process? The way your blood flows through your vessels and delivers oxygen to your cells and tissues will be reflected in your health, your appearance, and your brain function as the years roll by. What ultimately accelerates aging is your circulatory system.

Can you stop it, slow it, make old age easier to handle? Or have genetics already determined the answer in a sealed envelope? I believe the best answer to that question, your very best hope in aging gracefully, is to protect your circulatory system.

It is never too late to improve and restore your circulation. When your blood can't flow because of choices you've made or toxins you've invited into your blood vessels, your healthspan will be affected. Want to look good? Want to slow aging? Keep your blood vessels healthy. Study after study has shown that you can start at any age to reverse the damage that's been done to your circulation.

TIPS: *The following list includes noninvasive tests that can determine the health of your blood vessels.*
- *Lung function—at the frontline of the circulatory system, the lungs ensure that oxygen in the air gets into the bloodstream. Asthma, cystic fibrosis, emphysema, and chronic bronchitis can all interfere with oxygen entering our bodies. A pulmonary function test records the rate and amount you breathe in and out into a spirometer. A value less than 80 percent is abnormal.*
- *Blood sugar level (fasting blood sugar, hemoglobin A1c, fasting insulin level, LP-IR). All the test results should be evaluated together.*
- *Blood pressure—A measurement of less than 120/80 mm/Hg is ideal.*
- *Percentage body fat—More accurate than body mass index (BMI) because it measures fat content rather than muscle. Using calipers or bioelectrical impedance analysis or fat percentage scales.*
- *Exercise tolerance (stress test for the heart)—This is done on a treadmill wearing a heart monitor.*
- *Degree of inflammation (C-reactive protein and myeloperoxidase)—These blood tests can reveal inflammation, damage to blood vessels, and predicting cardiovascular disease.*
- *Cholesterol profile—Higher LDL level may represent higher state of inflammation if accompanied by low HDL level and translate into higher risk. Total cholesterol to HDL ratio should be below 5, but ideally, it should be*

below 3.5. And triglyceride to HDL should be below 2 to be at lower risk. An LDL subfraction test identifies the number and the size of the LDL particles.

- *Carotid intima media thickness (CIMT)—An ultrasound study that assesses the degree of atherosclerosis by measuring the wall thickness of the internal carotid artery, this is a noninvasive test done with an ultrasound probe on the neck. This test should be done for people who are generally older than forty-five to fifty.*
- *Vascular reactivity index—A noninvasive test that looks at the flexibility of blood vessels and involves a simple cuff on the arm for five minutes, a brisk temperature rebound measured at the fingertip is a sign of healthy and flexible vessels.*
- *Pulse wave velocity—This measures stiffness of a blood vessel.*

Chapter 6: Unleashing the Power of Our Circulation

So here we've come to the crux of it: The quality and length of your life begins and ends with the ability of your blood to deliver oxygen to your cells. Everything in our bodies relies on it, every disease we experience is affected by it, and our old age will be shaped by it. What we do and how well we do it is always a reflection of how our blood flows.

What are the most essential, simplistic ways to unleash the power of our circulation and live a long, healthy life?

At the core are food and exercise. Your choice of food, how much you eat, and how often you move are well within your control. It's a mind-set rather than a particular formula. Learn the skills and tools necessary to navigate your health. Without it, you are at the mercy of corporate marketers, big food and pharmaceutical companies, and healthcare providers who may be ill equipped.

It starts with your understanding that lifestyle choices *really* matter. Here are the surest ways to have your circulatory system work for you.

Eat right

Asking yourself how you've made choices about food in the past might help you as you seek to make better choices in the present and future. Here's a list of questions:

What is food to you? Is it a way to socialize and share or a symbol of love and security?
Is it a status symbol? A comfort or a necessity?
What role does nutrition play in your food choices?
What part does your culture play in your food choices—culture meaning what you learned to eat as a child or what is deemed socially admired or acceptable at this current moment in your life?
Is it based on affordability?
What about the size of your plate or the size of the drink you buy—the portion? How did you come to decide the right portion?
How did you begin to eat the foods you regularly partake in?
How did you choose the foods that fill your refrigerator, pantry, or grocery cart?
How did you decide what restaurants to go to or what to order?

Where did all these feelings you have about food come from? Is it hard to focus on nutrition when nutritional advice keeps on changing?
Do you buy things that sound healthy—yogurt and granola bars—only to hear later that they aren't healthy?
What if I told you that a great part of your eating habits is dictated by industry and economy and a biological craving you no longer really need?

The Western Diet

Today's Western diet consists of processed meats, white flour; high salt, high sugar, low fiber ingredients; while low in fruits, vegetables and whole grains. The Western diet is cheap and convenient and much of it is processed, which means it has been manipulated to have the right color, texture, and smell to make you crave it. Unfortunately, these foods are often high in calories while sorely lacking in nutrition. It makes us fat and sick, and slows our circulation.

Let's take a close look at a favorite appetizer and Super Bowl snack—the chicken wing. What's in it? Chicken fried twice and slathered in salty, sugary barbecue sauce and dipped in a ranch dressing that is full of calories. Tastes good? Of course. Fun American custom? Check. Good for you? Nope.

The Story of Bread

Let's analyze one of our favorite staple foods, one people have been enjoying for centuries—bread. Originally, the flour used in the bread was made by using whole grains, like wheat, and grinding them between two stones—the ground material would contain bran and germ in the wheat seed. But the bread was so dense it was hard to eat. So bread makers took out the bran and germ in the seed, which created white flour and softer bread. Flour mills were built, and it became quicker and more cost effective to make white flour (which also lasts longer on the shelves) and more white bread. But the softer, whiter bread lacked the nutrients, vitamins, and fiber from germ and bran. All that was left was refined carbohydrates, which break down into glucose quickly and spike blood sugar. This new, nutrition-less bread became a staple

[113]

We Westerners eat close to 1000 percent *more sugar* every day than
people did one hundred years ago. If you eat bread, white rice, pasta
or sauces or ketchup, you are eating sugar. And if you drink soda,
you're getting a huge dosage of sugar. While it varies depending on
where you live, it's pretty hard to get away from it.

In the parts of the world where people have the longest and
healthiest lives, what do they eat? Diets rich in plants and complex
grains but low in meat and virtually no added sugar or salt or foods
that have been manipulated. Guess what they don't have—high rates
of cancer, obesity, type 2 diabetes, and heart disease.

They aren't destroying their circulatory systems by causing
inflammation in their blood vessels. And they aren't destroying the
walls of their guts, allowing toxins to slip into the bloodstream—
because this is yet another result of a high-sugar diet filled with
highly processed food.

Leaky Gut
Your gut, where most of your immune system resides, is
the gatekeeper to your bloodstream and body, so it is
important to keep it healthy. Most toxins you consume
pass through the gut first. Some believe a diet that is high
in gluten, sugars, processed foods, and high-fructose corn
syrup can lead to leaky gut syndrome—so can antibiotics,
painkillers, and stress. In this condition, the lining of the
intestinal wall is damaged or inflamed by yeast or bad
bacterial growth. As a result, it becomes porous, which
allows germs, toxins, food particles, and other substances
to start slipping into the bloodstream. This can lead to
chronic inflammation and injury to blood vessels.
To protect your bloodstream, you must preserve nearly
one hundred trillion microorganisms (aka gut
microbiome) that live in your gut. They are assigned the

[114]

task of maintaining equilibrium in the intestine and aid in digestion. Your gut contains 80 percent of the body's immune system. You can start by not abusing antibiotics (which includes antibiotic fed meats), eating a whole-food diet rich in fiber, and minimizing stress. A key to combating damage to that intestinal lining is adding fermented foods like kimchi, yogurt, and sauerkraut to your diet. Fermented foods are probiotic, meaning that they contain ample amounts of good bacteria. Eating probiotic foods or supplements can promote a healthy gut.

Macronutrients and Micronutrients

Carbohydrates, fats, and proteins are all macronutrients, the structural and energy-giving caloric components of food. Micronutrients are the vitamins, minerals (trace elements), phytochemicals, and antioxidants that are essential for good health.

Processed foods usually have more macronutrients and fewer micronutrients. The processing strips the vitamins, minerals, and phytochemicals out of the food, so it will have a longer shelf life. Foods like cereals, breads, white rice, sweets, candy, and processed dairy products are high in calories but low in micronutrients.

The quality of the macro- and micronutrients depends on how and where natural food was raised or grown. Basically, you'd like your diet to be made up of 15–20 percent protein, 20–35 percent fat and 45–65 percent carbohydrates, plus plenty of micronutrients.

Protein

Every single cell in your body contains protein—the building block of life. The basic structure of protein is a chain of amino acids. It helps your body repair cells and make new ones. It is especially important for growth and development in the young and pregnant women. We need to consume essential amino acids, which our body cannot make. As we age, proteins are vital to keeping our muscle mass intact and maintaining our bone strength. Proteins in our bodies have many specific jobs, like catalyzing chemical reactions, aiding in communication between cells, or transporting molecules. When there is a shortage of fats or carbohydrates, proteins can be broken down and used, but since protein serves numerous functions in our body, it should be the last source of energy.

During digestion, protein in foods is broken down into amino acids that are used to build new proteins. You'll find amino acids in animal sources, such as meats, fish, eggs, and milk. These food sources also contain different amounts of fat and nutrients. Amino acids from protein are also found in plant sources such as soy, legumes, nut butter, and some grains like quinoa and wheat germ (hemp seeds provide complete essential amino acids). You can get all the protein you need without eating any animal products if you want to, although animal products are the most abundant source of protein. When consuming animal products, it's ideal to eat natural meats such as grass-fed beef, free-range chicken, and wild fish and to consume them with lots of vegetables to help with digestion.

Carbohydrates

There's a limit to how many carbs can be stored in the body at a time, so carbohydrates are the first nutrient the body uses for energy. Carbs from food are turned into either glucose or a sugar that is easily converted to glucose in small pieces, which can be absorbed through the small intestinal walls. Glucose passes through the liver and heads into the bloodstream, where it gets converted to energy by the cells. Cells prefer glucose, rather than fat, as their primary energy source.

Once the cells are full, the liver stores the leftovers as glycogen (about 400 calories) for snacks between meals and when blood glucose levels get low. Our muscles can also store up to 2000 calories as glycogen. Glucose that the liver and muscles can't hold gets turned into fat. When carbohydrates are scarce, the body starts running on fats—first fat in the diet, and then fat from your body where it has been stored.

Calorie wise, people should generally take in between 45 to 65 percent of their total calories in carbohydrates according to the National Institutes of Health. A diet of 1,800 calories would equal between 202 and 292 grams of carbs per day.

Simple versus complex carbohydrates

The difference between simple and complex has to do with how quickly the sugar can be absorbed or digested, which relates to chemical structure. Simple carbs contain just one or two sugars. Single sugars—like fructose, which is found in fruits and galactose, which is found in dairy products—are called monosaccharides. If the carb has two sugar molecules, like sucrose in table sugar or lactose in milk, they are known as disaccharides.

Processed and refined sugar found in candy, syrup, and sodas are loaded with simple carbs while lacking in fiber, vitamins, and minerals. Full of empty calories, they simply lead to weight gain and blood vessel damage.

Complex carbs come with fibers and starch, in addition to sugar, and they are known as polysaccharides. They are found in starchy foods like beans, peas, lentils, peanuts, corn, cereals, and whole grain breads.

So, here's the real difference between simple and complex: Simple carbs provide sudden, quick bursts of energy. They are quickly digested and absorbed, and if not used up immediately, they lead to sugar spikes and sugar highs, and can damage the blood vessels.

Complex carbs provide slow and sustainable energy with a gradual rise in blood sugar. Complex carbs from vegetables, fruits, and whole grains should be your main source of carbohydrates. When people talk about low-carb diets, what they really mean is a low-refined-carb diet. Eating complex carbohydrates is both healthy and necessary.

Fats

Trans fats, or the bad fats, are a byproduct of a process called *hydrogenation*. Hydrogenation is used to turn healthy oils into solids and to prevent them from becoming rancid. Healthy vegetable oils become unhealthy fats. On food label ingredient, this manufactured substance is typically listed as "partially hydrogenated oil." At first, these trans fats were used in solid margarines and vegetable shortening, but now they are used in processed cookies, pastries, and fast-food french fries.

Trans fats create inflammation and are linked to high blood cholesterol. Even consumption of small amounts of man-made trans fat daily can raise the risk of heart disease by 23 percent. There are no known health benefits to trans-fat, and they are slowly being removed from all food ingredients.

Good fats are fats your body needs to stay healthy. They are mainly found in vegetables, nuts, seeds, and fish. They come in two forms: monounsaturated and polyunsaturated fats.

[117]

Monounsaturated fats have a structure that keeps them liquid at room temperature. Good sources are olive oil, peanut oil, canola oil, as well as high-oleic safflower and sunflower oils. Avocados and most nuts are other great sources of monounsaturated fat. A study of Greece and other Mediterranean countries in the 1960s showed that Mediterranean people had a low rate of heart disease despite a high-fat diet. The main fat in their diet, however, was from olive oil, which contains mainly monounsaturated fat.

Although there's no recommended daily intake of monounsaturated fats, the Institute of Medicine recommends that our consumption of fats be from mono and polyunsaturated fats. That liquid cooking oil you put in a pan—corn oil, sunflower oil, safflower oil—contains mostly polyunsaturated fats. Other sources of polyunsaturated fats include nuts, leafy greens, and fatty fish. They are essential for building cell membranes and nerve coverings, and for blood clotting. The most common types are omega-3 fatty acids and omega-6 fatty acids. The American diet contains an overabundance of omega-6 and too little omega-3. Sources of omega-6 include most vegetable oils, such as corn, safflower, soybean, as well as poultry and eggs. Omega-3 fatty acids contain two important fats—EPA (eicosapentaenoic acid) and DHA (docosahexaenoic acid)—that are found in certain fish. ALA (alpha-linolenic acid) is another omega-3 that is found in plant sources, such as nuts and seeds. These are important in optimizing heart health.

Saturated fats are the most misunderstood fats and are found in animal meat, whole milk, eggs and other whole-milk dairy products, cheese, and many commercially prepared baked goods. They are also found in avocado, nuts, coconuts, and breast milk. While saturated fat is controversial, new research reviewing seventy-two studies found no link between saturated fats and heart disease—in fact, when consumed in moderate amounts, it can improve lipid profile.

To be clear, the cholesterol in our diets has almost no effect on our blood cholesterol levels and will not lead to heart disease.

Food Synergy over Nutritionism
Nutritional reductionism, or *nutritionism*, is the idea that food is simply the sum of its ingredients. It assumes that we can extract individual components from food and

reconstitute it in a food product to have the same beneficial effect. For instance, companies push the idea that adding vitamin C to a food through manufacturing will have the same benefit as eating an orange. It won't.

We look at food and try to break it down into key nutrients, but what are we missing? When we focus on individual nutrients instead of food as a whole, we are being nutritional reductionists. The government, food industry leaders, and pharmaceutical companies have espoused a reductionist theory, telling us what nutrients are essential by picking winners and losers. It has benefitted some businesses but harmed our bodies—as is evidenced by epidemic levels of obesity, insulin resistance, diabetes, heart disease, and cancer.

When a whole food is consumed, it has a synergistic effect, meaning the benefits of the nutrients altogether are greater than the sum of their individual parts. It's impossible to replicate food synergy in processed food.

Nutritionists know that people who eat whole food are healthier because they are consuming food rich in fiber, healthy fats, vitamins, minerals, and phytochemicals. Getting our nutrients from natural sources rather than supplements is always preferred.

TIPS: Don't eat food focused on each individual nutrient; use a holistic approach and consume whole foods as much as possible. Certain fad diets such as Pritikin, Paleo, and Alkaline diets have health benefits because they contain mostly unprocessed, whole foods, which are anti-inflammatory. Shop on the edges of the grocery store, where the whole foods are usually located. Look for foods as it exist in nature—not man-made—whether it's plant- or animal-based. Choose quality over quantity. Eat modest amounts of meat, lots of vegetables, whole grains, and fruits—a Mediterranean-style diet.

Eat Less

Back in 1917, President Woodrow Wilson's administration was worried about food shortages during World War I. A national campaign urged American citizens to sign pledge cards agreeing to not waste food and to "clean their plates" by eating everything on them. While the idea behind the doctrine was aimed at conserving food, it actually motivated people to eat more.

After World War II, President Truman resurrected the clean-the-plate idea. He persuaded Americans to finish their plates and send surplus food to starving people in Europe. Elementary schools started Clean Plate Clubs; eating every bite of lunch became a patriotic duty.

Still a vast majority of American parents are encouraging children to eat everything on their plates. A recent study from Cornell University concluded that clean-the-plate doctrine persists and influences eating behavior of children today. They showed when children were given larger bowls, they requested twice as much cereal, and the children who were told to clean their plates ate considerably more. Supersized portions coupled with a clean-the-plate mentality have been major contributors to overeating. A better practice, which centenarians in Okinawa, Japan, have followed for their whole lives is to put less on their plate and eat only until they are 80 percent full. This is called *hara hachi bu*. Eating to only satisfy hunger can be a difficult notion to comprehend. Complex issues involving emotion, addiction, psychology, and what's considered normal in our society play a role in eating disorders. But we must embrace eating less, because it can protect our blood vessels, keep us healthy, and allow us to live longer lives.

What does "eating less" mean exactly? While the medical community agrees that reduction in calories can slow aging, there aren't a lot of long-term studies on human beings. After all, telling people to simply eat less isn't a very profitable endeavor for food and drug companies, now is it?

Advocates of eating less call it *calorie restriction* and practice it at each meal. Many studies on restricting calories point to it as one of the most effective ways to slow aging and add to your healthy years. According to studies on nematodes, fruit flies, and rodents, even a modest reduction of calories can extend lifespan.

[120]

Two research projects into how rhesus monkeys (primates that closely resemble humans) respond to calories showed that eating fewer calories reduces the risks of chronic diseases that seem to go hand in hand with aging, while eating more had clear health consequences.

The main benefit of calorie restriction is making cells more sensitive to insulin, thereby decreasing blood sugar and leading to improved blood flow. Humans and animals that live long tend to have unusually low insulin levels, most likely because their cells are more responsive to the hormone insulin and therefore need less of it. Lower blood sugar is better for your circulation, reduces risk of diabetes, obesity, cardiovascular problems, neurodegenerative diseases, and even cancer. Calorie restriction also appears to reduce free radical formation, inflammation, and cellular stress.

But what does eating less look like? When done properly, each meal is full of nutritious whole food. It doesn't mean you have to feel deprived or look malnourished. It does involve reducing your calories by 10 to 25 percent of the standard American diet and making sure that your food intake is full of vitamins, minerals, and essential fatty acids. It takes time to reach your goal, and no one is advocating uncomfortable fasting. The original model for a calorie-restrictive diet came from the centenarians in Okinawa, Japan. They grew up on a diet that was 20 percent lower in calories than other Japanese. This Okinawan diet seemed to protect against heart disease, stroke, and cancer.

Fortunately, a number of studies have shown that *intermittent fasting* can produce many of the same health benefits as calorie restriction. Psychologically, this seems to be more doable—eating a normal amount followed by a fasting period. Scientists even favor this alternative approach over reducing calories because it can actually accelerate metabolism. Some people fast every other day, eating a normal amount of whole foods on the eating day. Others fast two days per week. If not eating for an entire twenty-four hours seems too difficult, there's an alternative.

A variation of intermittent fasting, called *time-restricted eating*, refers to eating during a compressed amount of time—let's say from 7:00 a.m. to 7:00 p.m. If you restrict your eating to a smaller window during the day—twelve to eight hours—your energy

[121]

metabolism improves. Even if you are eating the same amount of calories, this eating strategy will yield weight loss.

You can enjoy the same advantages that come from calorie restriction by consuming all your food in a twelve-hour period. Here's what happens: If you eat all day, your body can never burn off all the glycogen because it takes an average of eight to twelve hours to metabolize the sugar stored as glycogen. But in *time restricted eating*, your body is spending time in both a fed and a fasted state. During the fed state, you are consuming all the calories. When you switch over to the fasting state, your body runs out of glycogen and then begins to use fat as the energy source, giving your body time to lower blood sugar and insulin levels. A recent study found that average Americans spend nearly fifteen hours a day eating; that's five hours more each day compared to 1970.

Eating fewer calories and giving your body time to burn energy before it's turned into fat are two of the most beneficial changes you can make to protect your blood vessels and increase your healthy years.

TIPS: Many of us need to rethink the way we eat. Eating less may mean eating more food that make you feel full while containing less calories. Fruits and vegetables are generally high in water content, which provides volume and weight but not calories. For example, a whole grapefruit is 90 percent water and about 74 calories. One raw carrot is 88 percent water and about 25 calories. High fiber foods—whole grains, legumes, fruits, and vegetables—are low in calories, take longer to digest, and make you feel full longer.

Don't look at time-restricted eating as fasting but as a healthful eating schedule. Give yourself time to adjust to the new schedule. Have full and satisfying meals; then, do not eat for twelve hours, preferably beginning three hours before bedtime. I suggest 7:00 p.m. to 7:00 a.m. During this twelve-hour period, drink only water or tea and be sure not to eat. This allows the body to draw down sugar and insulin and start burning fat. Blood sugar will be lower and give you unexpectedly more energy. If you want to lose weight, you can compress the time even more to eight hours of eating by skipping breakfast (16/8 diet).

Move More

The first line of defense against circulation problems? Exercise. Here's why: Moving large muscles in our arms, legs, and hips in repetition makes us breathe faster and deeper, maximizing the amount of oxygen in our blood. Your heart will beat faster and harder, which increases blood flow to your entire body. Blood vessels will widen, more capillaries will open up, and new ones will form. It can even restore the flexibility of your blood vessels. Your skin and organs will glow as more oxygen is delivered to them. *Exercise is the best way to get oxygen into your body!*

Exercise plays a key role in the metabolism of sugar. During a workout, there is an increased uptake of sugar from the bloodstream into the muscles. A slight drop in the blood sugar mobilizes the glycogen (stored form of sugar) from both the liver and the muscles. Glycogen is the primary fuel source and it is quickly converted to sugar. Shortly after a workout, your muscles must replenish the depleted glycogen, and it gets it from the sugar in your blood. Exercise also turbocharges your insulin and dramatically improves insulin sensitivity for up to forty-eight hours. *Exercise is the best way to control your blood sugar level!*

Exercise activates an enzyme in the muscles and tissues called *AMPK* (*AMP-activated protein kinase*), which helps break down fats and sugar. Exercise also promotes the release of two specific neurotransmitters—serotonin and norepinephrine—reducing depression and stress, and lifting our mood. It even has a powerful anti-inflammatory effect on our bodies.

Studies show that exercise can keep you from gaining weight, help you lose weight, speed up your metabolism, increase your stamina, prevent viral illnesses, and reduce risks of obesity, heart disease, high blood pressure, insulin resistance, type 2 diabetes, metabolic syndrome, stroke, Alzheimer's disease, and cancer. During exercise, there is threefold increased production of brain-derived neurotrophic factor (BDNF)—BDNF is a key protein that is involved in protecting and maintaining the health of the brain. Weight-bearing exercise helps prevent osteoporosis. Even short bursts of hot, sweaty exercise (high intensity exercise) have been shown to help people of all shapes, sizes, and chronic-disease states live longer. So if you can, try to sweat. Move for sure—sweat if you can!

Unfortunately, in our everyday lives, we barely need to leave our houses anymore. Research at the library? That's what Google is for. Dating? Match.com. Banking? Just snap a picture of your check and deposit it. You can grocery shop, gift shop, have a meal catered, consult with your doctor, find out your medical history, watch the latest movies or a whole television series, play games, and go to college online. You don't even have to leave your house to have tea with your mother, conference with your child's teacher, or attend a meeting across the globe. You don't really have to get out of your seat if you don't want to.

And speaking of getting out of your chair—if you want, you can wear a bracelet that reminds you to move, tracks your every move, or tells you when you haven't moved. We've come to a point in our society where we have to be *reminded* to move, meaning a technology company is making money off a problem created largely by other technology companies.

Change is necessary. New ideas about eating and moving are required to combat our addictions to sugar and processed foods and leading sedentary lives.

If you need motivation, consider the help of a trainer, training apps, or DVDs—and be sure to look for resources that instruct on your form so you can exercise safely without injury and get the most benefits. Something as simple as joining a friend on a long walk or an exercise program can help you get started. Partnering with a group for a run or cycling is a great way to stay engaged and accountable. And for people who have physical limitations or are recovering from an injury, a physical therapist may be invaluable in helping to get back on their feet faster.

Exercise is not optional; it's crucial to your survival. And don't think you can't lose your ability to exercise. You can! Your bones can become brittle from osteoporosis, your joints can stiffen, and your muscles can shrink. And then what? Stretching and balancing—think Chinese tai chi—are important for keeping your joints supple. Weight training or resistance exercise is vital to maintaining your muscle mass, which helps to keep your bones strong and your spine stable and helps maintain your height. And the more muscle mass you have, the higher your metabolism. Since muscle is active and demands more energy than fat does, you will end up burning a lot more sugar. Be consistent in your workout routine; it can be difficult to restart.

One of my favorite tips on exercising comes from the pioneer of fitness himself, Jack LaLanne. "If something is important to you, schedule it!" He also wisely referred to our circulatory system as the "river of life." Many of the weight machines you see in today's gyms were invented by Jack for Olympic athletes, and he himself opened one of the nation's first gyms in 1936.

A typical day for Jack included:
- ninety minutes of weight training
- thirty minutes of swimming
- ten raw vegetables
- a late breakfast and an early dinner

Even at ninety-six, the age he was when he died of pneumonia, he was still incredibly healthy. Jack understood early on that sugar and processed food were bad for the body. As a teenager, after years of eating sugar and junk food, he attended a lecture on nutrition and gave it all up for good. Eventually, he became one of the first (and arguably the most famous) fitness advocates in the world. His efforts have helped to shape health and fitness in America.

> **TIPS:** *I am not telling you to go out and exercise like Jack because most of us can't do it. However, what is so remarkable about him is his devotion and consistency to maintaining a daily exercise habit. You must dedicate regular time and schedule it as an absolute, like making an appointment with the doctor. Make it a top priority. Schedule it. Write it in your calendar as an appointment you cannot miss.*
>
> *Start slow because you don't want to hurt yourself. If you are not used to regular exercise, it can be difficult at first. Don't be intimidated by others. Set achievable goals that can be done regularly. If you are used to sitting a lot, then stand up and stretch and walk around.*
>
> *If you don't like the gym, do other activities that will get your muscles moving, like gardening, cleaning cars, brisk walking,*

[125]

yoga, or playing sports with friends. Once you start, being
physically active will become a natural part of your life.

Be Better Informed

"Education is the most powerful weapon which we can use to change the world."

Nelson Mandela

Children's Education

It's critical to start at the beginning. How about starting with our littlest ones? First, the four core school subjects—math, English/language arts, science, and social studies—should become five: the fifth should be health education, including information about anatomy and physiology, physical activity, nutrition, family health and sexuality, community and environmental health, mental and emotional health, personal and consumer health, tobacco, drugs, and alcohol. It's essential that students understand how the choices they make can damage their bodies—and how much of this damage starts in their blood vessels. It should start in elementary school and continue through twelfth grade. Physical movement should be stressed for its health significance over its athletic or competitive value. Nutrition needs to be taught and supported by what's served in the school cafeterias.

Learning how the body works throughout a child's lifetime is as important as reading all the Roald Dahl books or understanding algebra. Learning about obesity, diabetes, and cancer is the first step in making good lifestyle choices. It's time we make movement and health part of the core curriculum for the next generation. Words like *inflammation, atherosclerosis,* and *blood flow* should be a part of the conversation we have with children when we talk about health. Arm them with the facts and encourage them to be responsible. Connect their dots to health! Teach anatomy and physiology to them and tell them how all the systems in our body, work together. Give them the vocabulary for their bodies.

Why don't we value our children's knowledge of nutrition, disease prevention, physical growth and development, reproduction, mental health, and drug and alcohol abuse issues? How many parents ask for a conference with the health education or physical education teachers? Why aren't life skills as essential as their academic skills?

[126]

Healthy habits and choices start early. Poor life choices in the early years can lead to bad habits for a lifetime and contribute to obesity, diabetes, heart problems, and cancer tomorrow.

Teaching children about health must be a top priority! Because let's be real: somebody is educating our children about food and not everybody who gets their attention has their health in mind. For the companies who make junk food, they look at children and see dollar signs.

TVs and Computers

Research in psychology revealed that children younger than eight, view food marketing as being truthful and unbiased. If children were to watch TV just two hours a day, they would be exposed to over 100 food advertisements a week—most of which advertised unhealthy products. There is incontrovertible evidence linking food marketing and children's food choices. A Yale University study published in January 2016 in the online journal *Obesity Reviews* found that visual food cues, such as food advertising, had similar effect as real food exposure, especially when it came to junk food[14]. The ads your kids see on TV and on the internet create powerful cravings for food that will lead to obesity, inflammation in their blood vessels, atherosclerosis, and potentially chronic illnesses like heart disease and cancer.

A separate study found that both children and adults were strongly influenced by food advertising: both groups consumed considerably more unhealthy snack foods while watching television[15]. Yet another study showed a direct correlation between the number of televisions in the house with obesity among children and adolescents. Don't think your children aren't already being educated about what to eat and drink. If they're watching television or shows on internet, they're most likely getting the wrong information.

Yes, that other babysitter, entertainer, and sometimes educator—the television—has been shown in study after study to be an important risk factor for obesity—Harvard researchers proved that over a quarter of a century ago[16]. So are the whole array of sedentary activities that are now part of our children's lives—including computers, phones, and in car rides; all that sitting time is bad for them. And yet today's kids spend over 44.5 hours a week in front of

[127]

a TV, phone, or computer screen. We need to instill in them a sense of "fit time"—playing in the park, walking, running, dancing, *moving*. Support for active lifestyles is vital and should come from education and policies made at the federal, state, and local levels, as well as within our own homes.

Medical Education

You know who else needs to have this information? Your doctors and nurses! They can't spend most of their time only treating the sick. Sure, people will get sick. But in many cases, there are suggestions or instructions medical professionals can give *before* someone gets sick that might have prevented the ailment. If we teach this to children, we must also teach it to medical professionals. Our medical schools and nursing schools must emphasize nutrition, lifestyle medicine, and environmental medicine—preventive and wellness medicine should be part of the core of medical education. Medical school and nursing school must teach healthcare providers to address the underlying causes of disease. Your doctor should be less disease focused than *you* focused, looking at you as a *whole person*, not just a disease state or individual parts. Your nurses and doctors should talk to you about your lifestyle choices and situations and point out how they can influence chronic disease.

Medical schools and nursing programs need to educate future medical professionals on how to create a partnership with patients. They need to teach doctors to help prevent chronic diseases by being aware and preventing environmental exposures to toxins and understanding aspects of modern lifestyles that are contributing to their occurrence today. Let's be sure our medical community is prepared to offer this type of functional medicine. This will require a curriculum change for all doctors, whether they specialize in medicine or surgery. Currently, medical students learn anatomy, physiology, and then pathology and pharmacology, and go straight into medicine and surgery. There's no room for prevention and lifestyle intervention. Doctors need to be clear—lifestyle choices affect a patient's blood flow. Blood flow affects overall health and disease.

When we think of preventive medicine today, we often think of tests like mammograms, pap smears, endoscopy, colonoscopy, CT scans, and heart stress tests. Those tests are helping to diagnose a disease early and save lives, but they aren't actually helping to *prevent* diseases. True preventive medicine is avoiding disease altogether. While traditional medicine has gotten better at treating acute problems like appendicitis, heart attack, and infectious disease, it's gotten worse at taking care of chronic conditions like diabetes, heart disease, and obesity. Prevention in addition to early diagnosis is an even more powerful form of medicine.

Who's to Blame?

Medical schools and residencies teach doctors how to care for sick people. After all, that's when people usually show up at a doctor's office or hospital, isn't it? Hospitals' revenue comes from people who are ill; they don't make money from healthy people. But what if financial incentives were offered to doctors and healthcare facilities to keep patients healthy and disease free?

Pediatrics is already on board with the idea of seeing patients before they become sick, but once we hit twenty, we're on our own. From twenty to fifty, average Americans are rather poor at keeping up with wellness visits. It's as if we finish our teens, and are "fully cooked," in no need of observation or care. Wrong.

Up until now, there's been a reluctance to embrace true preventive medicine because it has never been considered "real" medicine. "Real" medicine is treating pneumonia or cancer or a problem, so it's no surprise that most doctors' knowledge about nutrition—which is central to preventive care—is limited. Nobody ever bothered to teach them that optimizing nutrition helps prevent disease or that exercise is part of medicine. If you try to strike up a conversation with a doctor on lifestyle adjustments like exercise and nutrition, the conversation is usually limited because doctors don't know, haven't been taught to value, and can't discuss these important parts of your health.

You may be surprised that this was intentional, an outcome of a 1910 study of medical education called the Flexner Report, which many aspects of today's medical education and practice are based on. While the Flexner Report vastly improved medical education, it also led to the elimination of alternative approaches to medicine, like nutrition. Today's doctors use evidence-based medicine to deliver high-tech, quick, but less personal care and generally don't have the time or the knowledge to give tips about nutrition and prevention. Doctors rely on clinical research for evolving treatment plans. However, according to a former editor-in-chief of the *New England Journal of Medicine*, much of this research is flawed.

Doctors treat disease as though it is an all-or-none phenomenon. However, our health exists on a spectrum from healthy to a diseased state. We move along the spectrum, sometimes gradually. We should not wait until a full-blown disease strikes but instead treat any abnormal issues as soon as they arise, moving further from disease instead of closer to it. This is the essence of preventive medicine.

Andrew Weil, a Harvard-trained physician and advocate for integrative medicine, calls our "healthcare system broken and too dependent on expensive technology and pharmaceutical drugs that often cause as much harm as good". He funds programs to train doctors in integrative medicine, emphasizing "prevention, self-care, reliance on the body's innate healing capacity, and low-tech, low-cost interventions used in conjunction with conventional medicine". Treating the whole body, instead of just a part, is scientifically proven as an ideal way to deliver patient care. Our physicians should be fearless in treating patients this way. They shouldn't be afraid of naturopathy, acupuncture, homeopathy, herbalism, lifestyle counseling, chiropractic medicine, or faith healing—these methods of holistic medicine are not quackery. Take acupuncture, using pressure points to trigger nerve impulses that lead to muscle relaxation, release of chemicals (endorphins), and improved circulation. Or look at Chinese herbal medicine, which uses remedies that serve as blood thinners, antioxidants, or cancer fighters. Or what of hypnotherapy, which has been shown to help people quit smoking and change their eating habits? Research has shown that the connection between mind and body is a powerful tool, confirming the benefits of meditation, prayer, and yoga. Above all, today's healthcare provider must embrace nutritional counseling and the use of physical activity as an integral part of the treatment plan.

Here's another truth about modern medicine: Because of access to information through the internet, patients can discover an enormous amount of information regarding their health. And your doctor should be encouraging you to do just that—know about how

[130]

your body works and be proactive in taking care of yourself. This is the essence of wellness medicine!

Before rushing to medicate symptoms, we should find out what is causing them, because symptoms are merely signs of a breakdown in the system. So what's wrong with the system? Remember, the arrival of symptoms means problems in the body (and the circulatory system) have been going on for a long time. By the time symptoms show up, you're dealing with years of bad habits and cumulative damage. Maintenance is required on these bodies of ours, and where should we take them to keep them in tip-top shape if not our doctor's office? Doctors should become purveyors of health, rather than just those who treat the sick.

A wellness center will be a place where patients will remain fully engaged with physicians, nurses, nutritionists, nutritional counselors, and life coaches during their entire lives. Health will be monitored throughout a lifetime, instead of from prenatal to eighteen and then not again until fifty or so. Even when you're healthy, you'll be seen and advised by healthcare professionals to stay that way, and if you have problems brewing in your body that you don't know about, you'll find out in time to make the necessary changes. Social media can be a great way to keep patients connected and remind them of healthy habits. We need to build lots of these medical wellness centers both inside and outside of hospitals. Let's change the role of hospitals from just a place for sick people to a place for well people who need monitoring. Blood tests, physical exams, and noninvasive tests are essential tools for noticing issues before they get out of hand in our bodies.

TIPS: *Here's what you need to know about your own body:*
- *Everything in your body is connected. The multiple systems (circulatory, digestive, endocrine, immune, etc.) within your body interact with one another at all times to maintain homeostasis or the dynamic state of equilibrium. A breakdown in one part of the body will affect other parts.*
- *Disease is usually years in the making, caused by progressive damage to cells.*
- *Not being sick does not equate to being healthy. Don't be complacent!*

[131]

- *Diseases don't usually come with loud warning bells.*
- *If you have symptoms, they must be investigated promptly because they generally signal that a disease is more advanced.*
- *Abnormal blood tests and elevated blood pressure are important signs that trouble is brewing. Have them checked regularly and don't ignore the numbers as you wait for a full-blown problem. Get tested regularly and take action early.*
- *Medications often treat only the symptoms and not the cause.*
- *What you eat has a huge impact on your health.*
- *Lifestyle changes are difficult to make, but don't wait until it is too late.*
- *Look for doctors who have a nutritionist and a life coach in their offices, showing they are willing to both treat your symptoms and try to cure you.*
- *Everything you eat, breathe, or touch can end up in your bloodstream.*
- *There is a reason for everything that happens in our bodies.*
- *Chronic diseases arise as a consequence of our bodies' striving to protect themselves from injury.*
- *Most diseases occur from a breakdown in your circulatory system. To stay healthy, you should focus on optimizing your blood flow.*

Metformin

When the Food and Drug Administration (FDA) gave the go-ahead for the diabetes medication metformin to begin human trials in 2016 as a drug with antiaging potential, it was a first step towards the agency recognizing aging as a drug target (TAME study-Targeting Aging with Metformin[17]). Prior to that, the FDA had only allowed for drugs to treat specific diseases. So why metformin?

A cost-effective and widely prescribed diabetes drug used in Europe for more than sixty years and FDA approved in the United States since 1995, metformin has surprised scientists by seeming to extend the lives of diabetics who take it. A study from Cardiff University in the U.K. showed that diabetics taking metformin lived longer than people who didn't have diabetes. This was peculiar, since diabetes generally takes eight years off a person's life.

When metformin was given to mice, their physical performance improved on both speed and endurance tests. Their longevity increased by nearly 40 percent—the human equivalent of living to almost 120. Many hail metformin as the metabolic Holy Grail with a fountain-of-youth effect.

So how does it work? Back in medieval times, a flowering perennial herb known by various names including *goat's rue*, *false indigo*, and *French lilac* (rich in guanidine), was often given to treat frequent urination associated with the disease we know today as diabetes. The plant was also used during plague epidemics to promote perspiration in the sick. But it was always considered too toxic for clinical use.

Over many years and several starts and stops, researchers around the world came to realize that *biguanide* (derived from guanidine), the key ingredient in metformin is a voracious glucose eater and given the brand name Glucophage. It works by improving insulin sensitivity in the muscles and liver, increasing cells' ability to utilize glucose, decreasing glucose production by the liver, and decreasing the absorption of glucose from the intestine—all of which helped to keep blood sugar low. Metformin mimics some aspects of calorie restriction. Unlike other diabetic medications, people on metformin lost weight. It also activates AMPK, similar to effects of regular exercise. Additionally, a few studies have shown that metformin prevents cognitive decline, increases bone mineral density, reduces calcium deposits in the coronary arteries, and lowers the risk of Alzheimer's disease.

Some researchers describe a delicate and risky interaction in a cell's powerhouse (mitochondria) that makes them stronger. The body gets its energy from the mitochondria in each cell, which trigger small electric currents. This process generates highly reactive oxygen molecules (free radicals) that can be harmful to the body, damaging both cells and DNA. That's where metformin comes in. It decreases the number of reactive oxygen molecules.

More good news: metformin is extremely safe, and is very cheap. It could help many people who are not diabetic. As we age, our bodies have more difficulty processing sugar, yet we continue to consume high amounts of refined carbs, and lots of people suffer

[133]

from high blood sugar problems without realizing it. If their blood sugar is borderline normal or slightly elevated, then there is no current treatment for them. While the acceptable fasting blood sugar level is below one hundred, it should be lowered further to below ninety. Doctors might also utilize additional tests, such as hemoglobin A1c, insulin level, LP-IR, and glucose tolerance to check for excess sugar in the bloodstream.

The bottom line is that elevated sugar in the body *is poison to your blood vessels.* It inflames them, hardens them, blocks them from vasodilation, and limits delivery of oxygen to every cell in your body. Taking metformin briefly or long-term can help lower your blood sugar by making insulin more sensitive. Reduction in your blood sugar means less assault on your blood vessels, allowing more capillaries to open up. Cells will celebrate as they receive more oxygen.

Metformin is even involved in lipid metabolism by decreasing triglyceride production in your body. It can slow the number of harmful small, dense LDL made by the liver, further lowering the risk of heart disease.

It's already being heralded as a wonder drug that protects your circulation from the damaging powers of too much sugar and processed foods. Furthermore, independent of its sugar-lowering effect, metformin targets the mechanics of the smallest blood vessels and the capillaries to improve their function, boosting the blood flow. It may well become the first drug to fight aging, and the fact that the FDA has allowed it to be investigated as such certainly speaks to the direct link between circulation and aging.

And the good news doesn't stop here—metformin also fights cancer. What has become evident is that people who take metformin get 30 to 50 percent fewer cancers in almost every instance. Also, studies have noted that patients who developed cancer had much better survival rates if they were on metformin[18]. It lowers blood sugar and makes insulin more sensitive; it decreases free radical formation and reduces inflammation. Additionally, metformin stabilizes the abnormal blood vessel growth that is the hallmark of many cancers. *Metformin takes away sugar from those sugar-hungry cancer cells and delivers more oxygen where it is needed.*

It can also inhibit cancer cell growth and proliferation. It does this by reducing insulin and insulin-like growth factor (IGF-1). IGF-

1 is thought to be involved in the formation of many types of cancer and alters the metabolism of cancer cells. Metformin seems to show its potential as a drug for preventing cancer in diabetics, and promising results are beginning to surface in its use as anticancer agent in patients without diabetes.

TIPS: Consider taking metformin if you are over the age of fifty, even if you don't have a sugar problem. As we age, our bodies have more difficulty handling sugar and our pancreases are constantly stressed to make more insulin. Metformin can help stabilize our blood sugar levels, delaying the onset of diabetes. You may also experience some weight loss while taking metformin. If your sugar levels are higher than the normal range, start ASAP. Metformin can be taken safely even by people who are not diabetic. It will not cause a drop in your blood sugar to a dangerous level. For those who do not have a major sugar problem, 500 mg of metformin taken once a day is a good starting point and can be increased to 1000 mg (500 mg twice a day). But metformin is even more effective in those who are prediabetic or have insulin resistance. Starting metformin early will have a protective effect on the heart, decrease the chance of developing diabetes, and possibly lower your cancer risk. You should monitor your sugar level regularly by checking hemoglobin A1c, fasting blood sugar, and LP-IR, two to three times a year. Metformin can even reduce the insulin requirement for type 1 diabetics. Long-term use of metformin can lead to vitamin B_{12} deficiency, be sure to check your B_{12} level.

Reversing Disease
We tend to think disease is inevitable and accept it as part of the aging process. Pill organizers are just considered a common accessory for people over the age of sixty. But they don't have to be.

When you think of childhood disease, you usually think of asthma, strep throat, or leukemia. But the reality is that the diseases we think of as chronic diseases that usually affect adults are becoming more prevalent in children.

Nearly one-third of children are overweight or obese, which puts them at risk for developing diabetes, hypertension, and heart disease. Doctors are seeing diabetes more often in young people, and it can lower their life expectancy by seventeen years. The damage to the circulatory system is starting at a young age.

Since disease exists on a spectrum, you may have a problem well before your doctor decides to treat it. If you haven't yet met the criteria that define full-blown disease, you will be only observed. In reality, with early intervention, the disease progression can be halted.

Our healthcare providers chase disease symptoms instead of curing the core problems. In our society, we've accepted diseases as permanent and immovable fixtures. In many cases, diseases can be reversed. Yes, they may have started early. Yes, they may have taken years to build up to their current conditions. But we don't have to just accept them and throw up a desperate prayer when they are finally discovered. We can fight back. *Remember, hypoxia is the common thread among all chronic diseases.*

First, visualize this: There was a cell or cells that were not getting enough oxygen. Those cells began to breakdown and became diseased.

- Where does oxygen come from? Your blood.
- What do these cells need to heal? More oxygen.
- How do we do this? By restoring blood flow.

Medications might treat a certain symptom of a chronic disease or keep a disease at bay, but they don't cure it. So what does? According to a Scandinavian study published in 2006, *exercise* is more effective at reducing risk and treating type 2 diabetes than medication. Exercise has also been shown to treat metabolic syndrome, reduce the risk of heart and lung disease, and help normalize blood pressure. It has been shown to lower the incidence of all forms of arthritis. Being more active can actually stop diseases from progressing and can even heal them!

Lose weight—by any means, including diet change, lifestyle adjustment, gastric bypass, or lap-band surgery—and your blood pressure goes down. Shed fat and you reverse high blood pressure.

Stop smoking and *immediately* heart rate and blood pressure begin to normalize. Within a few hours, the level of carbon monoxide begins to decline and results in increased oxygen for the whole body.

Heart disease can be reduced and reversed by diet changes, according Dr. Caldwell Esselstyn, in his book *Prevent and Reverse Heart Disease*. More recent studies are showing that high amounts of added sugar in diet cause heart disease. Eliminate added sugar and you reduce heart disease.

Here's a hopeful little story from Down Under about how quickly diseases can be reversed.

Dr. Kerin O'Dea's experiment:
In 1980, ten aboriginal Australians with type 2 diabetes and metabolic disorder were living in an urban setting consuming a typical Western diet. They were taken back to the outback, where they originally lived, and ate what they could hunt and collect, which meant they were physically active and only ate wildlife and plants. There were no grocery stores or restaurants. In just seven weeks, they each lost about twenty pounds and most of their symptoms of diabetes and metabolic abnormalities were gone—their blood sugar went down, and their lipid profiles improved.

I'm not suggesting that you head out with a spear and start hunting bison, but there are basic changes that we can all make in our everyday lives.

I urge you to consider that the epicenter of health and aging lies in your circulatory system. All the diets and directives to move and exercise are calls to a greater purpose: Let it flow! Unimpeded, unobstructed, as fast or as slow as it is needed to get to any organ, tissue, and cell—Let it flow.

[137]

It's really that simple—blood flow and vessel health is at the heart of a healthy life. Early aging and chronic disease are symptoms of an unhealthy circulatory system. You own this system—not the drug companies or the food industry or even your doctor. I've given you a lot of scientific evidence of its significance to your overall health, but here's the big reveal:

You are the keeper of your circulatory system.

Yes, you are the owner and the guardian. No one can take that away from you, but you need to protect this magnificent machinery. As I have spoken with my family, friends, patients, and strangers, this message has resonated in some way with each one of them. We have been given this precious gift. Let's be good stewards of it.

Our circulatory systems hold the key to our national escalating healthcare crisis. If you think of it as your personal and national transport system, it seems wise that, as a large community, we should make changes to keep it flowing smoothly by making good food and movement everybody's business. Little things we do every day—eating sweets and processed foods or sitting instead of moving—affect our risk of chronic disease, death, and aging, as well as our nation's healthcare costs.

It's hard to think about being sick when you aren't sick or to imagine that your circulatory system may already be ailing because of unhealthy food choices or lack of exercise. It's hard but important to act sooner rather than later.

There's no magic bullet for aging well or staying healthy. It's an accumulation of many choices made every day over our lifetimes. But don't wait. As tennis pro Arthur Ashe once said, "Start where you are. Use what you have. Do what you can." It's an easy message, so simple it can get lost in all the confusion of diets, fad treatments, and talk of longevity research—move your blood; let it flow.

The truth is that inside of each one of us, there is a brilliantly designed system that we can take care of individually and by supporting one another. It has taken me four years of medical school, eight years of residency, and many years in practice and of lifestyle research to realize that our *circulatory system* is at the heart of our health and wellness.

[138]

Eat healthy and just enough. Move your body as often as you can. And don't forget to smile.

Let that blood flow!

Bibliography

Introduction

Jones, Casey M. "Measurement Science in the Circulatory System." Cell Mol Bioeng.2014 Mar; 7(1): 1-14.

Reiber, Carl L. "A Review of the Open and Closed Circulatory Systems: New Terminology for Complex Invertebrate Circulatory Systems in Light of Current Findings." Int J Zoology. Vol 2009 (2009), Article ID 301284, 8 pgs.

Lewis, Tanya. "Human Heart: Anatomy, Function and Facts." Live Science March 22, 2016.

Chapter 1: Understanding Our Circulation

Ribatti, Domenico." William Harvey and the Discovery of the Circulation of the Blood." J Angiogenes Res. 2009; 1:3.

Singer, CJ. "A Short History of Anatomy from the Greeks to Harvey." (1957). New York: Dover Publications.

Harvey, William. "On the Motion of the Heart and Blood in Animals." 1628. Translated, Revised, Edited by Alex Bowie. 1889.

Porter, R. "Blood and Guts: A Short History of Medicine." (2004). New York: W.W. Norton.

Allen, JP. "The Essential Guide to Egyptian Mythology." (2003). Oxford Guide. P. 28. Berkley.

Schultz Stanley. "William Harvey and the Circulation of the Blood: The Birth of a Scientific Revolution and Modern physiology." Physiology 2002 Oct; 17(5): 175-180.

Gregory, Andrew. "William Harvey." Encyclopedia Britannica.

Friedman, Meyer. "Medicine's 10 Greatest Discoveries." (1998). New haven, Conn: Yale University Press.

Aird, W.C. "Discovery of the Cardiovascular System: From Galen to William Harvey." J Thrombosis and Haemostasis. July 2011; 9: 118-129.

Pearce, JM. "Malpighi and the Discovery of Capillaries." Eur Neurol. 2007; 58 (4); 253-5.

Key Players

Encyclopedia Britannica. "Cellular Respiration." Encyclopedia Britannica. 2018.

Zimmerman, Jerry J. "Cellular Respiration." Pediatric Critical Care. 2011: 1058-1072.

Hoffman, Mathew. "Picture of Blood." Web MD. 2014

Informed Health Online. "What Does Blood Do?" U.S. National Library of Medicine. 2010 Jan 21. Cologne, Germany: Institute for Quality and Efficiency in Health Care (IQWiG).

American Society of Hematology. "Blood Basics." American Society of Hematology.

Conley, CL. "Blood-Biochemistry." Britannica.com

Alberts, B. "Blood Vessels and Endothelial Cells." Molecular Biology of Cells. 4th Edition. Garland Science. 2002.

Hadi AR Hadi. "Endothelial Dysfunction: Cardiovascular Risk Factors, Therapy, and Outcome." Vasc Health Risk Anag. 2005 Sep; 1(3): 183-198.

Rajendran, P. "The Vascular Endothelium and Human Diseases." Int J Biol Sci. 2013; 1057-1069.

[141]

Higashi, Y. "Endothelial Dysfunction and Hypertension in Aging." Hypertension Research. 35, 2012; 1039-1047.

Hadi AR Hadi. "Endothelial Dysfunction in Diabetes Mellitus." Vasc Health Risk Manag. 2007 Dec; 3(6) 853-876.

Sena, Cristina. "Endothelial Dysfunction-A Major Mediator of Diabetic Vascular Disease." BBA-Molecular Basis of Disease. 2013 Dec; 1832(12): 2216-2231.

Boos, CJ. "Circulating Endothelial Cells in Cardiovascular Disease." J Am Coll Cardiol. 2006 Oct 17; 48(8):1538-47.

Popkin, Barry M. "Water, Hydration and Health." Nutr Rev. 2010 August; 68(8): 439-458.

Jequier E. "Water as an Essential Nutrient: The Physiological Basis of Hydration." Eur J Clin Nutr. 2010; 64: 115-123.

Blood Flow

Pfitzner J. "Poiseuille and His Law." Anaesthesia, 1986; 31: 273-275.

Batchelor, GK. "An Introduction to Fluid Dynamics." (Cambridge Mathematical Library). Cambridge: Cambridge Univ Press. doi:10.1017/CBO9780511800955.

Landis E. "Poiseuille's Law and the Capillary Circulation." J Physiol. 1933 Jan;103: 432-443.

Skalak, R. "Poiseuille Medal Lecture. Capillary Flow: Past, Present, and Future." Biorheology. 1990; 27(3-4): 277-93.

Srivastava, A. "Principles of Physics in Surgery: The Laws of Flow Dynamics Physics for Surgeons-Part1." Indian J Surg. July 2009; 71: 182-187.

Jacob, Matthias. "Regulation of Blood Flow and Volume Exchange Across the Microcirculation." Critical Care. 2016; 20: 319.

Intaglietta, M. "Vasomotion and Flowmotion: Physiological Mechanisms and Clinical Evidence." Vasc Med Rev. 1990; 1: 101-112.

Siddiqui A." Effects of Vasodilation and Arterial Resistance on Cardiac Output." J Clin Experiment Cardiol. 2011; 2: 170.

Maiorana A. "Exercise and the Nitric Oxide Vasodilatory System." Sports Med. 2003; 33(14):1013-35.

Joyner MJ. "Nitric Oxide and Vasodilation in Human Limbs." J Appl Physiol. 1997 Dec; 83(6): 1785-96.

Jerca L. "Mechanism of Action and Biochemical Effects of Nitric Oxide". J Prevent Med. 2002; 10(2): 35-45.

Johnson, J. "Local Thermal Control of the Human Cutaneous Circulation." J Appl Physiol. 2010 Oct; 109(4): 1229-1238.

Charkoudian N. "Mechanisms and Modifiers of Reflex Induced Cutaneous Vasodilation and Vasoconstriction in Humans." J Appl Physiol. 2010 Oct; 109(4): 1221-1228.

Clifford, P. "Vasodilatory Mechanisms in Contracting Skeletal Muscle." J Appl Physiol. 2004. 97(1).

Altunkan S. "Arterial Stiffness Index as a Screening Test for Cardiovascular Risk." Eur J Intern Med. 2005 Dec; 16(80): 580-584.

Oliver J. "Noninvasive Assessment of Arterial Stiffness and Risk of Atherosclerotic Events." Arteriosclerosis, Thromb and Vasc Biol. 2003; 23: 554-566.

Ahluwalia, A. "Dietary Nitrate and the Epidemiology of Cardiovascular Disease: Report from a National Heart, Lung, and

[143]

Blood Institute Workshop." J Am Hear Assoc. 2016 Jul: 5(7) e003402.

Velmurugan, S. "Dietary Nitrates Improves Vascular Function in Patients with Hypercholesterolemia: A Randomized, Double-Blind, Placebo-Controlled Study." Am J Clin Nutr. 2016 Jan; 103(1): 25-38.

Lidder, S. "Vascular Effects of Dietary Nitrate (as found in green leafy vegetables and beetroot) Via the Nitrate-Nitrite-Nitric Oxide Pathway." Br J Clin Pharmacol. 2013 Mar; 75(3): 677-696.

Machha, A. "Dietary Nitrite and Nitrate: A Review of Potential Mechanisms of Cardiovascular Benefits." Eur J Nutr. 2011 Aug; 50(5): 293-303.

De Smet, S. "Nitrate Intake Promotes Shift in Muscle Fiber Type Composition During Sprint Interval Training in Hypoxia." Front physiol. June 2016; 7: 233.

Hoon, M. "The Effect of Nitrate Supplementation on Exercise Performance in Healthy Individuals." Int J Sport Nutr Exerc Met. 2013; 23: 522-532.

Bondonno CP. "Dietary Flavonoids and Nitrate: Effects on Nitric Oxide and Vascular Function." Nutr Res. 2015 Apr; 73(4): 216-235.

[1]Cassidy, A. "Dietary Flavonoid Intake and Incidence of Erectile Dysfunction." Am J Clin Nutr. 2016 Feb; 103(2): 534-541.

Hardening and Plaque Buildup

Stary, H. "A Definition of Advanced Types of Atherosclerotic Lesions and a Histological Classification of Atherosclerosis." Circulation. 1995 Sep 1; 92(5): 1355-74.

Hansson G. "The Immune Response in Atherosclerosis: A Double-Edged Sword." Nat Rev Immunology. 2006 July; 6: 508-519.

Braganza DM. "New Insights into Atherosclerotic Plaque Rupture." Postgrad Med J 2001; 77: 94-98.

Libby, P. "Atherosclerosis: The New View." Sci Am. 2002 May; 286 (5): 46-55.

Sangiorgi G. "Arterial Calcification and Not Lumen Stenosis is Highly Correlated with Atherosclerotic Plaque Burden in Humans." J Amer Coll Cardiol. 1998 Jan. Vol. 31(1): 126-133.

Leopold, JA. "Vascular Calcification: Mechanisms of Vascular Smooth Muscle Cell Calcification." Trends Cardiovasc Med. 2015 May; 25(4): 267-274.

Wilens, SL. "Evolution of Atherosclerotic Plaque." JAMA. 1964; 189(2): 167.

Libby P. "Inflammation and Atherosclerosis." Circulation. 2002; 105: 1135-143.

Packard R. "Inflammation in Atherosclerosis from Vascular Biology to Biomarker Discovery and Risk Prediction." Clin Chem. 2008 Jan; 54(1): 24-38.

Wong B. "The Biological Role of Inflammation in Atherosclerosis." Canadian J Cardiol. 2012 Nov; 28(6): 631-641.

Singh R. "Pathogenesis of Atherosclerosis: A Multifactorial Process." Exp Clin Cardiol. 2002 Spring; 7(1): 40-53.

Ritman, EL. "The Dynamic Vasa Vasorum." Cardiovasc Res. 2007 Sep 1; 75(4): 649-658.

Xu, J. "Vasa Vasorum in Atherosclerosis and Clinical Significance." Int J Mol Sci. 2015 May; 16(5): 11574-11608.

Huff, MW. "Can a Vascular Smooth Muscle—Derived Foam-Cell Really Change Its Spot?" Arterio Thromb Vasc Biol. 2015; 35: 492-495.

[145]

Kalampogias, A. "Basic Mechanisms in Atherosclerosis: The Role of Calcium." Med Chem. 2016; 12(2): 103-13.

Wang-Michelitsch, J. "Misrepair Mechanism in the Development of Atherosclerotic Plaques." Eprint. 2015 May. arXiv:1505.01289.

O'Rourke, C. "Calcification of Vascular Smooth Muscle Cells and Imaging of Aortic Calcification and Inflammation." J Vis Exp. 2016; (111): 54017.

Shanahan, CM. "Inflammation Ushers in Calcification." Circulation. 2007; 116: 2782-2785.

Van der Wal, AC. "Atherosclerotic Plaque Rupture-Pathologic Basis of Plaque Stability and Instability." Cardiovasc Research. 1999 Feb; 41(2): 334-344.

Neves, PO. "Coronary Artery Calcium Score: Current Status". Radiol Bras. 2017 May-Jun; 50(3): 182-189.

Lucas, A. "Atherosclerosis, Cancer, Wound Healing, and Inflammation." J Clin Exp Cardiology 3:e107, 2012.

Problems Can Begin Early in Life

Shah, P. "Screening Asymptomatic Subjects for Subclinical Atherosclerosis." J Amer Coll Cardiol. 2010 Jul. Vol. 56(2): 98-105.

Widimsky P. "Prevalence of Coronary Atherosclerosis in Asymptomatic Population."
Eur Heart J. 2000 Jan; 21(1) 13-4.

[2]Larose, E. "Young, Apparently Healthy—and at Risk of Heart Disease: New Study Pinpoints Hidden Thickening of the Arteries in Young Adults." Science daily. Oct 26, 2011. Heart and Stroke Foundation of Canada.

Joseph A. "Manifestations of Coronary Atherosclerosis in Young Trauma Victims-An Autopsy Study." J Am Coll Cardiol. 1993; 22(2): 459-467.

Strong, JP. "Prevalence and Extent of Atherosclerosis in Adolescents and Young Adults." JAMA. 1999; 281(8): 727-735.

Strong, JP. "Early Lesions of Atherosclerosis in Childhood and Youth: Natural History and Risk Factors." J Am Coll Nutr. 1992 Jun 11; Suppl: 51S-54S.

Surgeon's Perspective

Taylor, GI. "The Vascular Territories (Angiosomes) of the Body: Experimental Study and Clinical Applications." JPRAS. 1987 Mar; 40(2): 113-141.

Hosein, RC. "Postoperative Monitoring of Free Flap Reconstruction: A Comparison of External Doppler Ultrasonography and the Implantable Doppler Probe." Plast Surg. 2016 Spring; 24(1): 11-19.

Athletes

Aubrey, J. "Lance Armstrong Confesses to EPO and Blood Doping." Cycling News. January 13, 2013.

Robinson, N. "Erythropoietin and Blood Doping." Br J Sports Med. 2006 July; 40(Suppl 1): i30-i34.

Bryner, J. "What is Blood Doping?" Live Science. January 3, 2013.

Lundby, C. "The Evolving Science of Detection of Blood Doping." Br J Pharmacol. 2012 Mar; 165(5): 1306-15.

Robinson, R. "The Ethiopia/Kenya Running Phenomenon." Running Times. March 19, 2014.

Wilber, RL. "Kenya and Ethiopian Distance Runners: What Makes Them So Good." Int J Sports Physiol Perform. 2012 Jun; 7(2): 92-102.

Bailey, DM. "Physiological Implications of Altitude Training for Endurance Performance at Sea Level: A Review." Br J Sports Med 1997; 31: 183-190.

Wolski, LA. "Altitude Training for Improvements in Sea Level Performance." Sports Medicine. 1996 Oct; 22(4): 251-263.

Desplanches, D. "Muscle Tissue Adaptations of High-Altitude Natives to Training in Chronic Hypoxia or Acute Normoxia." J Appl physiol. November 1996. Vol.81(5): 1946-1951.

Alexander, B. "The Secret Science of Novak Djokovic's Training Pod." Outsideonline. Feb 20, 2015.

[3]Taddei S. "Physical Activity Prevents Age-Related Impairment in Nitric Oxide Availability in Elderly Athletes." Circulation. 2000 June 27; 10(25): 2896-901.

Weil. A. "Three Breathing Exercises and Techniques." DrWeil.com.

Emergencies

James, G. "New York Killings Set a Record, While Other Crimes Fell in 1990." New York Times. April 23, 1991.

Clark, R. "The Golden Hour and the Difference Between Life and Death." KevinMD.com. February 9, 2011.

Pham, H. "Faster On-Scene Times Associated with Decreased Mortality in Helicopter Emergency Medical Services Transported Trauma Patients." Trauma Surg Acute Care Open. 2017; 2: e0001.

El Sayad, M. "Recent Advances of Hemorrhage Management in Severe Trauma." Emerg Med Int. 2014; 2014: 638956.

Chapter 2: How Our Circulation Impacts the Body

<u>Skin</u>

Amirlak, B. "Skin Anatomy." Medscape. Updated Nov. 29, 2017.

Cable, NT. "Unlocking the Secrets of Skin Blood flow." J Physiol. 2008 May 1; 572(pt3): 613.

Roberts, MF. "Control of Skin Circulation During Exercise and Heat Stress." Med Sci Sports. 1979 Spring; 11(1): 36-41.

Sonksen J. "Circulation of the Skin." Current Anesth Crit Care. 1999 April; 10(2): 58-63.

Charkoudian, N. "Skin Blood Flow in Adult Thermoregulation: How It Works, When It Does Not, and Why." Mayo Clin Proc. 2003 May; 78(5): 603-12.

Gunin, AG. "Age-Related Changes of Blood Vessels in the Human Dermis." Adv Gerontol. 2015 Apr; 5(2): 65-71.

Nosarev, AV. "Exercise and NO Production: Relevance and Implications in the Cardiopulmonary System." Front Cell Dev Biol. 2014; 2: 73.

Crane, JD. "Exercise-Stimulated Interleukin-15 is Controlled by AMPK and Regulates Skin Metabolism and Aging." Aging Cell. 2015 Aug; 14(4): 625-634.

Black, MA. "Exercise Prevents Age-Related Decline in Nitric Oxide Mediated Vasodilator Function in Cutaneous Microvessels." J Physiol. 2008 Jul 15;586(14): 3511-24.

Britt, R. "Exercise Linked to Reduced Skin Cancer Risk." Live Science. May 13, 2006.

[149]

Conney, AH. "Inhibition of UVB-Induced Nonmelanoma Skin Cancer: A Path from Tea to Caffeine to Exercise to Decreased Tissue Fat." Top Curr Chem. 2013; 329: 61-72.

Schagen, S. "Discovering the Link Between Nutrition and Skin Aging." Dermatoendocrinol. 2012 Jul 1; 4(3): 298-307.

Tarnofsky, MA. "Endurance Exercise Rescues Progeroid Aging and Induces Systemic Mitochondrial Rejuvenation in mtDNA Mutator Mice." PNAS. 2011.

Tarnofsky, MA. "Exercise as Countermeasure for Aging: From Mice to Humans". American Medical Society for Sports Medicine. 2014.

Tarnofsky MA. "Endurance Exercise Prevents Premature Aging: Mcmaster Study."
February 21, 2011.

Cals-Grierson, MM. "Nitric Oxide Function in the Skin." Nitric Oxide. M2004 Jun; 10(4): 179-93.

Heart

Taylor, AM. "Cardiac Anatomy Revisited." J Anat. 2004 Sep; 205(3): 159-177.

Swanoski, MT. "Knowledge of Heart Attack and Stroke Symptomology: A Cross-Sectional Comparison of Rural and Non-Rural US Adults." BMC Public HeaLTH. 2012. 12:283.

Mayo Clinic Staff. "Coronary Artery Disease." Overview. Mayo Clinic Website.

Wee, Yong. "Medical Management of Chronic Stable Angina." Aust Prescr. 2015 Aug; 38(4): 131-136.

Davies, SW. "Clinical Presentation and Diagnosis of Coronary Artery Disease: Stable Angina." Brit Med Bull. 2001 Oct; 59(1): 17-27.

[150]

Lichtman, JH. "Symptom Recognition and Healthcare Experience of Young Women with Acute Myocardial Infarction." Circulation: Cardiovascular Quality and Outcomes. 2018 Feb; 11(2).

Quah J. "Knowledge of Signs and Symptoms of Heart Attack and Stroke Among Singapore Residents." Biomed Research Int. 2014; 2014: 572425.

Liver

Sear. J. "Anatomy and Physiology of the Liver." Baill Clin Anesthesiology. 1992 Dec; 6(4): 697-727.

Eipel, C. "Regulation of Hepatic Blood Flow: The Hepatic Arterial Buffer Response Revisited." World J Gastroenterol. 2010 Dec; 16(48): 6046-6057.

Ebrahimi, H. "New Concepts on Pathogenesis and Diagnosis of Liver Fibrosis.; A Review article." Middle East J Dig Dis. 2016 Jul; 8(3): 166-178.

Dysom, JK. "Republished: Non-Alcoholic Fatty Liver Disease: A Practical Approach to Treatment." BMJ Journals. 2015 Feb: 91(1072).

Neuschwander-Teteri, BA. "Non-Alcoholic Fatty Liver Disease." 2017; 15(45).

Suzuki, T. "Hypoxia and Fatty Liver." World J Gastroenterol. 2014 Nov; 20(412): 15087-15097.

Suk, KT. "Staging of Liver Fibrosis or Cirrhosis: RThe Role of Hepatic Venous Pressure Gradient Measurement." World J Hepatol. 2015 Mar; 7(3): 607-615.

Nath, B. "Hypoxia and Hypoxia Inducible Factors: Diverse Roles in Liver disease." Hepatology. 2012 Feb; 55(2): 622-633.

[151]

Hall, P. "What is the Real Function of the Liver 'Function' Tests?" Ulster Med J. 2012 Jan; 81(1): 30-36.

Kumar, M. "Is Cirrhosis of the Liver Reversible?" Indian J Pediatr; 2007 Apr; 74(4): 393-399.

Takahashi, H. "Correlation Between Hepatic Blood Flow and Liver Function in Alcoholic Cirrhosis." World J Gastroenterol. 2014 Dec; 20(45): 17065-17074.

Mental Health

Purves D. "The Blood Supply of the Brain and the Spinal Cord." Neuroscience. 2nd Edition. 2001. Sinauer Associates.

Jones, O. "The Arterial Supply to the Central Nervous System". TeachMeAnatomy. January 2, 2018.

Detre, JA. "Migraine with Aura is Associated with an Incomplete Circle of Willis: Results of a Prospective Observational Study." PLOS One 8(7) e71007. July 26, 2013.

Doll, DN. "Cytokines: Their Role in Stroke and Potential Use as Biomarkers and Therapeutic Targets." Aging Dis. 2014 Oct; 5(5): 294-306.

Ahn, MJ. "The Effects of Traumatic Brain Injury on Cerebral Blood Flow and Brain Tissue Nitric Oxide Levels and Cytokine Expression." J Neurotrauma. 2004 Oct; 21(10): 1431-42.

Varatharaj, A. "The Blood-Brain Barrier in Systemic Inflammation." Brain, Behavior, and Immunity. 2017 Feb; 60: 1-12.

Smith, RS. "The Immune-Brain Connection." Cytokines and Depression. Chapter 3. 1997.

Silva B. "Memory Deficit Associated with Increased Brain Pro-Inflammatory Cytokine Levels and Neurodegeneration in Acute Ischemic Stroke." Arq Neuro-Psiquiatr. 2015 Aug; 73(8).

Singh, B. "A Prospective Study of Chronic Obstructive Pulmonary Disease and the Risk for Mild Cognitive Impairment." JAMA Neurol. 2014 May; 71(5): 581-8.

Ishizaki, J. "Changes in Regional Cerebral Blood Flow Following Antidepressant Treatment in Late-Life Depression." Int j Geriatr Psychiatry. 2008 Aug; 23(8): 805-11.

Nobler, MS. "Effects of Medications on Cerebral Blood Flow in Late-Life Depression." Curr Psych Reports. 2002 Jan; 4(10): 51-58.

Querido JS. "Regulation of Cerebral Blood Flow During Exercise." Sports Med. 2007; 37(9): 765-82.

Ide K. "Cerebral Blood Flow and Metabolism During Exercise." Prog Neurobiol. 2000 Jul; 61(4): 397-414.

Zhang, P. "Early Exercise Improves Cerebral Blood Flow Through Increased Angiogenesis in Experimental Stroke Rat Model." J NeuroEng Rehab. 2013;10:43.

[4]Craft LL. "The Benefits of Exercise for the Clinically Depressed." Prim Care Comp J Clin Psychiatry. 2004; 6(3): 104-11.

Sharma, A. "Exercise for Mental Health." Prim Care Comp J Clin Psychiatry. 2006; 8(2): 106.

Blumenthal JA. "Is Exercise a Viable Treatment for Depression?" ACSMs Health Fit J. 2012 Jul/Aug; 16(4): 14-21.

Babyak, M. "Exercise Treatment for Major Depression: Maintenance Therapeutic Benefit at 10 Months." Psychosomatic Med. 2000 Sep/Oct; 62(5): 633-638.

Blumenthal, JA. "Exercise and Pharmacotherapy in the Treatment of Major Depressive Disorder." Psychosom Med. 2007;69(7): 587-596.

[153]

Barnes, JN. "Sugar Highs and Lows: The Impact of Diet on Cognitive Function." J Physiol. 2012 Jun15; (12): 2831.

Chang, CY. "Essential Fatty Acids and Human Brain." Acta Neurol Taiwan. 2009 Dec; 18(4): 231-241.

Dyall, SC. "Long-Chain Omega-3 Fatty Acids and the Brain: A Review of the Independent and Shared Effects of EPA, DPA, and DHA." Front Aging Neurosci. 2015; 7: 52.

Penckofer, S. "Vitamin D and Depression: Where is All the Sunshine?" Issues Ment Health Nurs. 2010 Jun; 31(6): 385-393.

Bedrosian, TA. "Timing of Light Exposure Affects Mood and Brain Circuits." Translational Psychiatry. 7, e1017 (2017).

Parry, BL. "Light Treatment of Mood Disorders." Dialogues Clin Neurosci. 2003 Dec; 5(4): 353-365.

Vision

Jager, RD. "Age-Related Macular Degeneration." N Engl J Med 2008;3582606-2617.

Burgansky-Eliash Z. "Retinal Blood Flow Velocity in Patients with Age-Related Macular Degeneration." Curr. Eye Res. 2014 Mar; 39(30: 304-311.

Boltz, A. "Choroidal Blood Flow and Progression of Age-Related Macular Degeneration in the Fellow Eye in Patients with Unilateral Choroidal Neovascularization." Invest Ophthalmol Vis Sci. 2010 Aug; 51(8): 4220-5.

Grunwald, JE. "Reduced Foveolar Choroidal Blood Flow in Eyes with Increasing AMD Severity." Invest Ophthalmol Vis Sci. 2005 Mar; 46(3): 1033-8.

Wong, I. "Prevention of Age-Related Macular Degeneration." Int Ophthalmol. 2011 Feb; 31(1); 73-82.

Rasmussen HM. "Nutrients for the Aging Eye." Clin Interv Aging. 2013; 8: 7451-748.

Duh, EJ. "Diabetic Retinopathy: Current Understanding, Mechanisms, and Treatment Strategies." JCI Insight. 2017 Jul; 2(14): e93751.

Shah, AR. "Diabetic Retinopathy: Research to Clinical Practice." Clin Diabestes Endocrinol. 2017; 3(9).

Lee, R. "Epidemiology of Diabetic Retinopathy, Diabetic Macular Edema and Related Vision Loss." Eye Vis (Lond). 2015; 2: 17.

Hair

Wester RC. "Minoxidil Stimulates Cutaneous Blood Flow in Human Balding Scalps: Pharmacodynamics Measured by Laser Doppler Velocimetry and Photopulse Plethysmography." J Invest dermatol. 1984 May; 82(5): 515-7.

Messenger AG. "Minoxidil: Mechanisms of Action on Hair Growth." Brit J Dermatol. 2004; 150(2).

Yano, K. "Control of Hair Growth and Follicle Size by VEGF-Mediated Angiogenesis." J Clin Invest. 2001 Feb. 15; 107(4) 409-17.

Detmar, M (Mass General Hospital). "Blood Vessels Hold Key to Thicker Hair Growth." ScienceDaily. Feb. 19, 2001.

Yamada, T. "Male Pattern Baldness and its Association with Coronary Heart Disease: A Meta-Analysis." BMJ Open. 2013; 3(4): e002537.

[5]Klemp, P. "Subcutaneous Blood Flow in Early Male Pattern Baldness." J Invest Derm. 1989 May; 92(5): 725-726.

Goldman, BE. "Transcutaneous PO_2 of the Scalp in Male Pattern Baldness: A New Piece of the Puzzle." Plast Reconstr Surg. 1996 May; 97(6): 1109-1116.

Orasan, MS. "Hair Loss and Regulation Performed on Animal Models." Clujul Med. 2016; 89(3): 327-334.

Koyama, T. "Standardized Scalp Massage Results in Increased Hair Thickness by Inducing Stretching Forces to Dermal Papilla Cells in the Subcutaneous Tissue." Eplasty. 2016; 16 e8.

Dhurat R. "Response to Microneedling Treatment in Men with Androgenetic Alopecia Who Failed to Respond to Conventional Therapy." Indian J dermatol. 2015 May-Jun; 60(3): 260-263.

Dhurat, R. "A Randomized Evaluator Blinded Study of Effect of Microneedling in Androgenetic Alopecia: A Pilot Study." Int J Trichology. 2013 Jan-May; 5(1):6-11.

Sexual Function

Solomon, H. "Erectile Dysfunction and the Cardiovascular Patient: Endothelial Dysfunction is the Common Denominator." Heart. 2003; 89: 251-53.

Kaya, C. "Is Endothelial Function Impaired in Erectile Dysfunction Patients?" Int J Impot Res. 2006 Jan-Feb; 18(1): 55-60.

Masters, WH. "Human Sexual Response." Published 1966.

Francis, SH. "Sidenafil: Efficacy, Safety, Tolerability and Mechanism of Action in Treating Erectile Dysfunction." Expert Opin Drug Metab Toxicol. 2005 Aug; 1(2):283-93.

Maharaj, C. "Effects and Mechanism of Action of Sidenafil Citrate in Human Chorionic Arteries." Reprod Biol Endocrinol. 2009; 7:34.

Musicki, B. "Endothelial Nitric Oxide Synthase Regulation in Female Genital Tract Structures." J Sex Med. 2009 Mar 1;6 (S3Proceedings): 247-253.

Strong Muscles

Mcphron, AC. "Increasing Muscle Mass to Improve Metabolism." Adipocyte. 2013 Apr 1; 2(2): 92-98.

Srikanthan, P. "Relative Muscle Mass is Inversely Associated with Insulin Resistance and Prediabetes. Findings from the Third National Health and Nutrition Examination Survey." J Clin Endocrinol Metab. 2011 Sep; 96(9): 2898-903.

Gornik, H. "Peripheral Arterial Disease." Circulation. 2005; 111: e169-e172.

Kamel, HK. "Sarcopenia and Aging." Nutr Rev. 2003 May; 61(5pt 1): 157-67.

Ramasamy, SK. "Blood Flow Controls Vascular Function and Osteogenesis." Nat Commun. 7. 2016; Article Number: 13601.

Vogt, MT. "Bone Mineral Density and Blood Flow to the Lower Extremities: The Study of Osteoporotic Fractures." J Bone Min Res. 1997; 122(2): 283.

Kim, S. "The Association Between the Low Muscle Mass and Osteoporosis in Elderly Korean People." J Korean Med Sci. 2014 Jul; 29(7): 995-1000.

Ferrucci, L. "Interaction Between Bone and Muscle in Older Persons with Mobility Limitations." Curr Pharm Des. 2014; 20(19): 3178-3197.

Ginaldi, L. "Osteoporosis, Inflammation and Ageing." Immun Ageing. 2005; 2:14.

Williams, D. "Acclimation During Space Flight: Effects on Human Physiology." CMAJ. 2009 Jun 23; 180(13): 1217-1323.

Demontiero, O. "Aging and Bone Loss: New Insights for the Clinician." Ther Adv Musculoskelet Dis. 2012 Apr; 4(2): 61-76.

Olin, JW. "Peripheral Artery Disease: Current Insight into the Disease and its Diagnosis and Management." Mayo Clin Proc. 2010 Jul; 85(7): 678-692.

Ernst EE, "Intermittent Claudication, Exercise, and Blood Rheology." Circulation. 1987; 76: 1110-1114.

Bailey, MA. "Clinical Assessment of Patients with Peripheral Arterial Disease." Semin Intervent Radiol. 2014 Dec; 31(4): 292-299.

Hamburg, NM. "Exercise Rehabilitation in Peripheral Arterial Disease: Functional Impact and Mechanism of Benefits." Circulation. 2011 Jan 4; 123(1): 87-97.

Chapter 3: Factors That Influence Our Circulation

Inflammation

Hunter, Philip. "The Inflammation Theory of Disease." EMBO Rep. 2012 Nov; 13(11): 968-970.

Straub, RH. "Chronic Inflammatory Systemic Diseases: An Evolutionary Trade-Off Between Acutely Beneficial but Chronically Harmful Programs." Evol Med Pub Health. Vol. 2016; 1:37-51.

Kidd, BL. "Mechanisms of Inflammatory Pain." Brit J Anaesth. 2001 Jun; 87(1): 3-11.

Granger DN. "The Microcirculation and Inflammation: Modulation of Leukocyte-Endothelial Cell Adhesion." J Leukoc Biol. 1994 May; 55(5): 662-75.

Emanuela, F. "Inflammation as a Link between Obesity and Metabolic Syndrome." J Nutr Metabol. 2012; 2012: 476380.

Granger, DN. "Capillary Perfusion". Inflammation and Microcirculation." San Rafael: Morgan Claypool Life Sciences; 2010. Chapter 5, Capillary Perfusion.

Ye, J. "Adipose Tissue Vascularization: Its Role in Chronic Inflammation." Curr Diab Rep. 2011 Jun; 112(3): 203-210.

Eardley, KS. "The Role of Capillary Density, Macrophage Infiltration and Interstitial Scarring in the Pathogenesis of Human Chronic Kidney Disease." Kidney Inter. 2008 Aug; 74(4): 495-504.

Sullivan, GW. "The Role of Inflammation in Vascular Diseases." J Leukoc Biol. 2000 May; 67(5): 591-602.

Nolte, D. "Functional Capillary Density: An Indicator of Tissue Perfusion?" Int J Microcirc Clin Exp. 1995 Sep-Oct; 15(5): 244-9.

Tsai, AG. "Capillary Flow Impairment and Functional Capillary Density." Int J Microcirc Clin Exp. 1995 Sep-Oct; 15(5): 238-43.

Minihane, AM. "Low Grade Inflammation, Diet Composition and Health: Current Research Evidence and Its Translation." Br J Nutr. 2015 Oct; 114(7): 999-1012.

Ricker MA. "Anti-Inflammatory Diet in Clinical Practice: A Review." Nutr Clin Practice. 2017 Jun; 32(3): 318-325.

Esposito, K. "Diet and Inflammation: A Link to Metabolic and Cardiovascular Diseases." Eur Heart Journ. 2006 Jan; 27(1): 15-20.

Olivera, Cd. "Toothbrushing, Inflammation, and Risk of Cardiovascular Disease: Results from Scottish Health Study." BMJ. 2010 May; m340: c2451.

Anatoliotrakis N. "Myeloperoxidase: Expressing Inflammation and Oxidative Stress in Cardiovascular Disease." Curr Top Med Chem. 2013; 13(2): 115-138.

Ridker, PM. "Comparison of C-Reactive Protein and Low-Density Lipoprotein Cholesterol in the Prediction of First Cardiovascular Events." N England J Med. 2002 Nov; 347: 1557-1565.

Simmonds, S. "Testing for C-Reactive Protein May Save Your Life." Lifeextension. May 2014,

Salazar J. "C-Reactive Protein: Clinical and Epidemiological Perspectives." Cardiol Research Pract. 2014: 1-11.

Cholesterol

Steinberg, D. "Hypercholesterolemia and Atherosclerosis in Humans: Causally Related?" Science Direct. 2007. Lipid Hypothesis.

Fernandez, C. "Effects of Distal Cholesterol Biosynthesis Inhibitors on Cell Proliferation and Cell Cycle Progression." J Lipid Res. 2005 May; 46(5): 920-9.

Ravnskov, U. "The Fallacies of the Lipid Hypothesis." Scand Cardiovasc J. 2008 Aug; 42(4): 236-9.

Univ. of Washington. "Cholesterol, Lipoproteins and the Liver." University of Washington Online.

Wikipedia. "Low-Density lipoprotein." Wikipedia.

Timesofindia. "The Function of Cholesterol in the Body." Timesofindia.com Nov. 6, 2017.

Enig, MG. "The Importance of Cholesterol on the Body". Know Your Fats: The Complete Primer for Understanding the Nutrition of Fats, Oils and Cholesterol." Bethesda Press 2001.

Koly, D. "How Do LDL and HDL Differ Structurally and Functionally?" Livestrong.com. Aug 14, 2017.

Nayeri, H. "LDL Fatty Acids Composition as a Risk Biomarker of Cardiovascular Disease." Artery Research. 2017 Dec.; 20: 1-7.

Perlmutter, D. "LDL is Your Friend." DavidPerlmutter MD Empowering Neurologist.

Mcevoy, M. "Cholesterol is Powerfully Anti-Inflammatory and Prevents Free Radicals." Metabolic Healing. July 20, 2011.

Waterham, HR. "Defects of Cholesterol Biosynthesis." Science Direct. 2006 Oct; 580(23); 5442-5449.

Pejic, RN. "Familial Hypercholesterolemia." Ochsner J. 2014 Winter; 14(4): 669-772.

Sircus. "Treat the Inflammation Not the Cholesterol." DrSircus. July 17, 2015.

Weil, A. "High Cholesterol." Weil Andrew Weil, MD.

Mercola JM. "Cholesterol Isn't the Problem in Heart Disease; Inflammation Is." Mercola.com; Sept 13, 2017.

Hyman, M. "Why Cholesterol May Not be the Cause of Heart Disease." Dr. Hyman.com/blog/2010/05.

Ravnskov, U. "High Cholesterol May Protect Against Infections and Atherosclerosis". QJM: Int J Med. 2003 Dec; 96(12): 927-934.

Herron, KL. "High Intake of Cholesterol Results in Less Atherogenic Low-Density Lipoprotein Particles in Men and Women Independent of Response Classification." Metabolism. 2004 Jun; 53(6): 823-30.

Kwiterovich, PO. "The Metabolic Pathways of High Density Lipoprotein, Low Density Lipoprotein, and Triglycerides: A Current Review." Am J Cardiol. 2000 Dec 21; 86(12A): 5L-10L.

Zhang, Y. "Systemic Inflammatory Markers are Closely Associated with Atherogenic Lipoprotein Subfractions in Patients Undergoing Coronary Angiography." Mediators Inflamm. 2015; 235742.

Parthasarathy, S. "Oxidized Low-Density Lipoprotein." Methods Mol Biol. 2010; 610: 403-417.

Mitra, S. "Oxidized Low-Density Lipoprotein and Atherosclerosis Implications in Antioxidant Therapy." Am J Med Sci. 2011 Aug; 342(2): 135-42.

Gao, S. "Association Between Circulating Oxidized Low-Density Lipoprotein and Atherosclerotic Cardiovascular Disease." Chronic Dis Trans Med. 2017 Jun; 3(2): 89-94.

Nelson, RH. "Hyperlipidemia as a Risk Factor for Cardiovascular Disease." Prim care. 2013 Mar; 40(1): 195-211.

Goldstein, J. "The LDL Receptor and the Regulation of Cellular Cholesterol Metabolism." J Cell Sci. 1985: 131-137.

Adams, DD. "The Great Cholesterol Myth; Unfortunate Consequences of Brown and Goldstein's Mistake." QJM:Int J Med. 2011 Oct; 104(10): 867-70.

Sobal, G. "Why is Glycated LDL More Sensitive to Oxidation than Native LDL? A Comparative Study." Prostaglandins Leukol Essent Fatty Acids. 2000 Oct; 63(4): 177-86.

Younis, N. "Glycation as an Atherogenic Modification of LDL." Curr Opin Lipidol. 2008 Oct; 19(5): 552.

Health.gov. "2015-2020 Dietary Guidelines for Americans." Health.gov. Dec 2015.

Brody, J. "What's New in the Dietary Guidelines." New York Times. January 18, 2016.

Ravnskov, U. "Lack of an Association on an Inverse Association Between Low- Density Lipoprotein Cholesterol and Mortality in the Elderly: A Systematic Review." BMJ Open. 2016; 6: e010401.

Kendrick, M. "Should Women be Offered Cholesterol Lowering Drugs to Prevent Cardiovascular Disease? No." BMJ. 2007: 334.

Curfman, G. "Risks of Statin Therapy in Older Adults." JAMA Intern Med. 2017; 177(7): 966. doi:10.1001/jamainternmed. 2017.1457

Weverling-Rijinsburger, AW. "Total Cholesterol and Risk of Mortality in the Oldest Old". Lancet. 1997 Oct 18; 350:1119-23.

Berkrot, B. "FDA Adds Diabetes, Memory Loss Warnings to Statins." Reuters.Feb 28, 2012.

Cederberg, H. "Increased Risk of Diabetes with Statin Treatment is Associated with Impaired Insulin Sensitivity and Insulin Secretion: A 6 Year Follow-Up Study of the METSIM Cohort." Dibetologia. 2015 May; 58(5): 1109-17.

Fdanews. "FDA Mandates New Safety Warnings for Statin Drugs Due to Risks of Memory Loss, Diabetes and Muscle Pain." FDA.NEWS. May 6, 2016.

Ganji, SH. "Niacin and Cholesterol: Role in Cardiovascular Disease (Review)." J Nutr Biochem. 2003 Jun; 14(6): 298-305.

Blake, GJ. "Are Statins Anti-Inflammatory?" Curr Control Trials Cardiovasc Med. 200; 1(3): 161-165.

Superko, HR. "Is it LDL Particle Size or Number that Correlates with Risk for Cardiovascular Disease." Curr Atheroscler Rep. 2008 Oct; 10(5): 377-85.

Ambrosch, A. "LDL Size Distribution in Relation to Insulin Sensitivity and Lipoprotein Pattern in Young and Healthy Subjects." Diabetes Care. 1998 Dec; 21(12): 2077-84.

Allaire, Janie. "LDL Particle Number and Size and Cardiovascular Risk: Anything New Under the Sun". Curr Op Lipidology. 2017 Jun; 28(3): 261-66.

Millan, J. "Lipoprotein Ratios: Physiological Significance and Clinical Usefulness in Cardiovascular Prevention." Vasc health Risk Manag. 2009; 5: 757-65.

Ivanova, EA. "Small Dense Low-Density Lipoprotein as Biomarker for Atherosclerotic Disease." Oxidat Med Cell Longevity. 2017 (2017), Article ID 1273042, 10 pages.

Choi, CU. "Statins Do Not Decrease Small, Dense Low–Density Lipoprotein." Tex Heart Inst. J. 2010; 37(4): 421-428.

Couillar, C. "Effects of Endurance Exercise Training on Plasma HDL Cholesterol Levels Depend on Levels of Triglycerides." Atheroscler Thromb Vasc Biol. 2001; 21: 1226-1232.

Wang, L. "Effect of a Moderate Fat Diet with and Without Avocados on Lipoprotein Particle Number, Size and Subclasses in Overweight and Obese Adults: A Randomized, Controlled Trial". J Am heart Assoc. 2015 Jan; 4(1): e001355.

Garoufi, A. "Plant Sterols-Enriched Diet Decreases Small, Dense LDL-Cholesterol Levels I Children with Hypercholesterolemia: A Prospective Study." Ital J Pediatr. 2014 May 3; 40:42.

Sugar

O'Connor, A. "How the Sugar Industry Shifted Blame to Fat." New York Times. Sept. 12, 2016.

Kearns, CE. "Sugar Industry and Coronary Heart Disease Research: A Historical Analysis of Internal Industry Documents." JAMA Intern Med. 2016 Nov 1; 176(11): 1680-1685.

McGrandy, RB. "Dietary Fats, Carbohydrates and Atherosclerotic Vascular Disease." N Engl J Med. 1967 Jul 27; 277(4): 186-92.

Shuto, Yuki. "Repetitive Glucose Spikes Accelerates Atherosclerosis Formation in C57BL/6 Mice." PLOS one. Aug 27, 2015.

Cavalot, F. "Postprandial Blood Glucose is a Stronger Predictor of Cardiovascular Events than Fasting Blood Glucose in Type 2 Diabetes Mellitus, Particularly in Women: Lessons from the San Luigi Gonzaga Diabetes Study." J Clin Endo Metabol. 2006 Mar; 91(3): 813-819.

Ceriello, A. "Postprandial Hyperglycemia and Diabetes Complications." Diabetes. 2005 Jan; 54(1): 1-7.

O'Keefe, JH. "Dietary Strategies for Improving Post-Prandial Glucose, Lipids, Inflammation, and Cardiovascular Health." J Am Coll Cardiol. 2008 Jan 22; 51(3): 249-55.

Yagihashi, S. "Mechanism of Diabetic Neuropathy: Where are We Now and Where to Go?" J Diabetes Investig. 2011 Jan; 245(2): 18-32.

Singleton, JR. "Increased Prevalence of Impaired Glucose Tolerance in Patients with Painful Sensory Neuropathy." Diabetes Cadre. 2001; 24(8): 1448-1453.

Summer, CJ. "The Spectrum of Neuropathy in Diabetes and Impaired Glucose Tolerance." Neurology. 2003; 60: 108-111.

Amagada, J. "Are You Non-Diabetic? Your After-Meal Blood Sugar Spikes may be Killing You Softly." The drjoe.com.

[165]

Hoffman-Snyder, C. "Value of the Oral Glucose Tolerance Test in the Evaluation of Chronic Idiopathic Axonal Polyneuropathy." Arch Neurol. 2006; 63: 1075-1079.

Jenkins, D. "Glycemic Index: Overview of Implications in Health and Disease." Am J Clin Nutr. 2002 Jul; 76(1): 266S-273S.

Radulian, G. "Metabolic Effects of Low Glycemic Index Diets." Nutr Journal. 2009; 8:5.

Stein, N. "Leading Sources of Added Sugar in the American Diet." Chron.com.

Ruff, JS. "Human-Relevant Levels of Added Sugar Consumption Increase Female Mortality and Lower Male Fitness in Mice." Nature Communications. 2013 Aug; 4: 2245.

Blaisdell, AP. "Food Quality and Motivation: A Refined Low-Fat Diet Induces Obesity and Impairs Performance on a Progressive Ratio Schedule of Instrumental Lever pressing in Rats." 2014; 128:220 DOI.

Hyman, M. "The Not-So-Sweet Truth about High Fructose Corn Syrup." Huffington Post. The Blog 5/13/2011.

Duffey KJ. "High-Fructose Corn Syrup: Is This What's for Dinner?" Am J Clin Nutr. 2008 Dec; 88(6): 1722S-1732S.

Lakhan, SE. "The Emerging Role of Dietary Fructose in Obesity and Cognitive Decline." Nutr J. 2013; 12:114.

Avena, NM. "Evidence for Sugar Addiction: Behavioral and Neurochemical Effects of Intermittent, Excessive Sugar Intake." Neurosci Biobehav Rev. 2008; 32(1): 20-39.

DiNicolantonio, JJ. "Sugar Addiction: Is it Real? A Narrative Review." Br J Sports Med. 2017 Aug 23.

Lenoir, M. "Intense Sweetness Surpasses Cocaine Reward". PLOS one. 2007 August. https://doi.org/10.1371/journal. Pone. 0000698.

Schroeder, J "Student-Faculty Research Suggests Oreos can be Compared to Drugs of Abuse in Lab Rats." Connecticut College. 2013.

Sharma A. "Artificial Sweeteners as a Sugar Substitute: Are They Safe?" Indian J Pharmacol. 2016 May-Jun; 48(3): 237-240.

Swithers, SE. "Artificial Sweeteners Produce the Counterintuitive Effect of Inducing Metabolic Derangements." Trends Endocrinol Metab. 2013 Sep; 24(9): 431-4541.

Alexander, S. "How Much Sugar is in Your Alcohol?" The Telegraph.October 134, 2015.

Colditz, GA. "Alcohol Intake in Relation to Diet and Obesity in Women and Men." Am J Clin Nutr. 1991 July; 54(1): 49-55.

Toffolo, MCF. "Alcohol: Effect on Nutritional Status, Lipid, Profile and Blood Pressure." J Endo Metabol. 2012 Dec; 2(6): 205-211.

Sacks, DB. "Measurement of Hemoglobin A1c." Diabetes Care. 2012 Dec; 35(12): 2674-2680.

Ikeda, F. "Haemoglobin A1c Even Within Non-Diabetic Level is a Predictor of Cardiovascular Disease in a General Japanese Population: The Hisayama Study." Cardiovac Diabetol. 2013 Nov 7; 12:164.

Selvin, E. "Glycemic Control and Coronary Heart Disease Risk in Persons With and Without Diabetes: The Atherosclerosis Risk in Communities Study." Arch Intern Med. 2005 Sept 12; 165(16): 1910-6.

Brambilla, P. "Normal Fasting Plasma Glucose and Risk of Type 2 Diabetes." Diabetes care. 2011 Jun; 34(6): 1372-1374.

Sacks, DB. "A1C Versus Glucose Testing: A Comparison." Diabetes Care. 2011 Feb.; 34(2): 518-523.

Florkowski, C. "HbA1c as a Diagnostic Test for Diabetes Mellitus-Reviewing the Evidence." Clin Biochem Rev. 2013 Aug; 34(2): 75-83.

Whitbread, D. "Top 10 Foods Highest in Sugar (To Limit or Avoid)." MyFoodData.

Jamers, Maia. "Safe Toothpaste Guide." Gimme the Good Stuff. July 7, 2016.

Smoking

Bergen, A. "Cigarette Smoking." J Nat Canc Inst. 1999 Aug; 91(16): 1365-1375.

Talhout, R. "Hazardous Compounds in Tobacco Smoke." Int J Environ Res Public Health. 2011 Feb; 8(2): 613-628.

Rabinoff, M. "Pharmacological and Chemical Effects of Cigarette Additives." Am J Public Health. 2007 Nov; 97(11): 1981-1991.

Cheng, T. "Chemical Evaluation of Electronic Cigarettes." BMJ Journals. 2012 Sep; 23(2).

Suter, TW. "Cardiovascular Effects of Smoking Cigarettes with Different Nicotine Deliveries." Psychopharmacology. 1983 May; 80(2): 106-112.

Papathanasiou, G. "Effects of Smoking on Cardiovascular Function: The Role of Nicotine and Carbon Monoxide". Health Science Journal.

Vineis, P. "Tobacco and Cancer: Recent Epidemiological Evidence." J Nat Canc Inst. 2004 Jan; 96(2): 99-106.

American Cancer Society. "Deciding to Quit Smoking and Making Plan." American Cancer Society.

American Cancer Society. "Quitting Smoking: Help for Cravings and Tough Situations." American Cancer Society.

Gordon, DL. "The 23 Best Ways to Quit Smoking." Readers Digest. Stealth Health (book).

Processed Food

Mercola, J. "7 Worst Ingredients in Food." Mercola:Take Control of Your health. Mercola.com.

Weaver, CM. "Processed Foods: Contributions to Nutrition." Am J Clin Nutr. 2014 Jun; 99(1): 1525-1542.

Steele, EM. "Ultra-Processed Foods and Added Sugars in the Diet: Evidence from a Nationally Representative Cross-Sectional Study." BMJ Open. 2016; 6(3): e009892.

National Research Council Committee on Diet, Nutrition, and Cancer. "Diet, Nutrition, and Cancer: Directions for Research." National Academies Press; 1983. 8, Food Additives. Contaminants, Carcinogens, and Mutagens.

Santarelli, RL. "Processed Meat and Colorectal Cancer: A Review of Epidemiologic and Experimental Evidence." Nutr Canc. 2008; 60(2): 131-144.

Joseph, M. "11 Harmful Food Additives Hiding in Processed Food." Nutrition Advance. January 13, 2017.

Nicole, W. "Secret Ingredients: Who Knows What's in Your Food?" Environ Health Perspect. 2013 Apr; 12(4): a126-a133.

Kobylewski, S. "Toxicology of Food Dyes." Intern J Occupat Environ Health. 20134 Nov; 18(3): 220-246.

Dwivedi, K. "Genetic Damage Induced by a Food Coloring Dye (Sunset Yellow) on Meristematic Cells of Brassica Campestris L." J Environ Public Health. 2015, Article ID 319727, 5 pages.

Mepham, B. "Food Additives: An Ethical Evaluation." Br Med Bulletin. 2011 Sep; 99(1): 7-23.

Physicians for Social Responsibility. "Toxic Chemicals in Our Food System." PSR.org.

Uribarri, J. "Advanced Glycation End Products in Foods and a Practical Guide to Their Reduction in the Diet." J Am Diet Assoc. 2010 Jun; 110(6): 911-16. e12.

Goldin, A. "Advanced Glycation End Product: Sparking the Development of Diabetic Vascular Injury." Circulation. 2006; 114: 597-605.

Tamanna, N. "Food Processing and Maillard Reaction Products: Effect on Human Health and Nutrition." Int J Food Sci. 2015(2015).

O'Connor, A. "So Will Processed Meat Give You Cancer?" The New York Times. Oct 31, 2015.

Stress

Ranabir, S. "Stress and Hormones." Indian J Endocrinol Metab. 2011 Jan-Mar; 15(1): 18-22.

Sanchez, O. "Acute Stress-Induced Tissue Injury in Mice: Differences Between Emotional and Social Stress." Cell Stress Chaperones. 2002 Jan; 7(1): 36-46.

Alkadhi, K. "Brain Physiology and Pathophysiology in Mental Stress." ISRN Physiology. 2013; 2013: 23 pages.

Nabi, H. "Increased Risk of Coronary Heart Disease Among Individuals Reporting Adverse Impact of Stress on their Health: The

Whitehall II Prospective Cohort Study." Eur Heart J. 2013 Sep; 34(34) 2697-2705.

Muldoon, MF. "Acute Cholesterol Responses to Mental Stress and Change in Posture." Arch Intern Med. 1992 Apr; 152(4): 775-80.

Assadi, S. "What are the Effects of Psychological Stress and Physical Work on Blood Lipid Profiles?" Medicine. 2017 May; 96(18): e6816.

Goyal, N. "Non-Diabetic and Stress Induced Hyperglycemia in Orthopedic Practice What Do We So Far?" J Clin Diag Res. 2014 oct; 8(10): LH01-03.

Dimsdale, JE. "Psychological Stress and Cardiovascular Disease". J Am Coll Cardiol. 2008 Apr; 51(13) 1237-1246.

Schneiderman, N. "Stress and Health: Psychological, Behavioral, and Biological Determinants." Annu Rev Clin Psychol. 2005; 1: 607-628.

McEwen, B. "Stress and Your Health." J Clin Endo Metab. 2006 Feb; 91(2): E2.

Moyer, AE. "Stress-Induced Cortisol Response and Fat Distribution in Women." Obes Res. 1994 May; 2(3): 255-62.

Bose, M. "Stress and Obesity: The Role of the Hypothalmic-Pituitary-Adrenal Axis in Metabolic Disease." Curr Opin endocrinol Diabetes Obes. 2009 Oct; 16(5): 340-46.

Abel, EL. "Longevity of Major League Baseball Players." Res Sports Med. 2005 Jan-Mar; 13(1): 1-5.

Hoge, EA. "Randomized Controlled Trial of Mindfulness Meditation for Generalized Anxiety Disorder: Effects on Anxiety and Stress Reactivity." J Clin Psychiatry. 2013 Aug; 74(8): 786-792.

Woodyard, Catherine. "Exploring the Therapeutic Effects of Yoga and its Ability to Increase Quality of Life." Int J Yoga. 2011 Jul-Dec; 4(2): 49-54.

Varvogli, L. "Stress Management Techniques: Evidence–Based Procedures that Reduce Stress and Promote Health." Health Science Journal.

Brower, V. "Mind-Body Research Moves Towards the Mainstream." Embo rep. 2006. Apr; 7(4): 358-361.

Chapter 4: Diseases of Our Circulation

<u>High Blood Pressure</u>

Giles, TD. "Definition and Classification of Hypertension: An Update." J Clin Hypertension. 2009 Nov; 11(11): 611-614.

Carretero, O. "Essential Hypertension-Part I: Definition and Etiology." Circulation. 2000; 101: 329-335.

Lionakis, N. "Hypertension in the Elderly." World J Cardiol. 2012 May; 4(5): 135-147.

Renna, NF. "Pathophysiology of Vascular Remodeling in Hypertension." Int J Hypertension. 2013; (2013): 7 pages.

Mayet, J. "Cardiac and Vascular Pathophysiology in Hypertension." Heart. 2003 Sep; 89(9): 1104-1109.

Mitchell, GF. "Arterial Stiffness and Hypertension." Hypertension. 2014; 64: 13-18.

Antonios, TF. "Microvascular Rarefaction in Hypertension-Reversal or Over-Correction by Treatment?" Am J Hypertension. 2006 May; 19(5): 484-485.

Sabino, B. "Effects of Antihypertensive Drugs on Capillary Rarefaction in Spontaneously Hypertensive Rats: Intravital

Microscopy and Histologic Analysis." J Cardiovasc Pharmaacol. 2008 Apr; 51(4): 402-9.

Mayet, J. "Cardiac and Vascular Pathophysiology in Hypertension." Heart. 2003 Sep; 89(9): 1104-1109.

Cheng, C. "Functional Capillary Rarefaction in Mild Blood Pressure Elevation." Clin Transl Sci. 2008 May; 1(1): 75-79.

Mourad, JJ. "Is Hypertension a Tissue Perfusion Disorder? Implications for Renal and Myocardial Perfusion." J Hypertens Suppl. 2006 Aug; 24(5): S10-6.

Levy, B. "Importance of Improving Tissue Perfusion During Treatment of Hypertension." J Hypertens Suppl. 2006 Aug; 24(5): S6-9.

Feihl, F. "Hypertension: A Disease of the Microcirculation." Hypertension. 2006; 48: 1012-1017.

Strauer, BE. "ACE-inhibitors and Coronary Microcirculation." Basic Res Cardiol. 1993; 88 Suppl 1: 97-106.

Gupta, R. "Strategies for Initial Management of Hypertension". Indian J Med Res. 2010 Nov; 132(5): 531-542.

Agabiti-Rosei, E. "Structural and Functional Changes of the Microcirculation in Hypertension: Influence of Pharmacological Therapy." Drugs. 2003; 63 spec no. 1: 19-29.

Levy BI. "Impaired Tissue Perfusion." Circulation. 2008; 118: 968-976.

[6]Mozaffarian, D. "Heart Disease and Stroke Statistics—2015 Update: Report from the American heart Association." Dec 17, 2014. Circulation. Doi: 10.1161/CIR.0000000000000152.

Diabetes

American Diabetes Association. "Diagnosis and Classification of Diabetes Mellitus." Diabetes Care. 2010 Jan; 33(Suppl 1): S62-69.

Goldenberg, R. "Definition, Classification and Diagnosis of Diabetes, Prediabetes and Metabolic Syndrome." Canadian J Diabetes. 2013 Apr; 37(Suppl)10: S8-11.

Ozougwu, JC. "The Pathogenesis and Pathophysiology of Type 1 and Type 2 Diabetes Mellitus." Academic Journals. 2013 Sep. 4(4): 46-57.

Beckman, JA. "Diabetes and Vascular Disease: Pathophysiology, Clinical Consequences, and Medical Therapy: Part II." Eur Heart J. 2013 Aug; 34(31): 2444-2452.

Dokken, BB. "The Pathophysiology of Cardiovascular Disease and Diabetes: Beyond Blood Pressure and Lipids." Diabetes Spectrum. 2008 Jul; 21(3): 160-165.

Wei, X. "De Novo Lipogenesis Maintains Vascular Homeostasis Through Endothelial Nitric Oxide Synthase (eNOS) Palmitoylation." J Biol Chem. 2011 Jan; 286(4): 2933-2945.

Mainous III, AG. "Prediabetes Diagnosis and Treatment in Primary Care." J Am Board Fam Med. 2016 Mar-Apr; 29(2): 283-285.

Stokes, A. "Deaths Attributable to Diabetes in the United States: Comparison of Data Sources and Estimation Approaches." PLoS. 2017; 12(1): e0170219.

Wu, Y. "Risk Factors Contributing to Type 2 Diabetes and Recent Advances in the Treatment and Prevention". Int J Med Sci. 2014; 11(11): 1185-1200.

[7]Stokes, A. "Deaths Attributable to Diabetes in the United States: Comparison of Data Sources and Estimation Approaches." PLoS ONE 12(1): e0170219. https://doi.org/10. 1371/journal.pone.0170219.

Wilcox, Gisela. "Insulin and Insulin Resistance." Clin Biochem Rev. 2005 May; 26(2): 19-39.

Kahn, BB. "Obesity and Insulin Resistance." J Clin Invest. 2000; 106(4): 473-481.

Bessesen, DH. "The Role of Carbohydrates in Insulin Resistance." Journal Nutr. 2001 October; 131(10): 27782S-2786S.

Utzschneider, KM. "The Role of Insulin Resistance in Nonalcoholic Fatty Liver Disease." J Clin Endocrinol Metab. 2006 Dec 1; 91(12): 4753-4761.

Howard, BV. "Insulin Resistance and Lipid Metabolism." Am J Cardiol. 1999 Jul; 84(1A): 28J-32J.

Hardy, OT. "What Causes the Insulin Resistance Underlying Obesity?" Curr Opin Endocrinol Diabetes Obes. 2012 Apr; 19(2): 81-87.

Nilson, G. "Waist Circumference Alone Predicts Insulin Resistance as Good as the Metabolic Syndrome in Elderly Women." Eur j Int Med. 2008 Nov; 19(7): 520-526.

Lustig, RH. "The Cholesterol and Calorie Hypotheses are Both Dead—It is Time to Focus on the Real Culprit: Insulin Resistance". 14 Jul 2017. Pharmaceutical J.

Huang, Y. "Association Between Prediabetes and Risk of Cardiovascular Disease and All Cause Mortality: Systematic Review and Meta-analysis." BMJ. 2016; 355: i5953.

[8]Pai, JK. "Hemoglobin A1c is Associated With Increased Risk of Incident Coronary Heart Disease Among Apparently Healthy, Nondiabetic Men and Women." J Am Heart Assoc. 2013 Apr; 2(2): e000077.

Al-Goblan, AS. "Mechanism Linking Diabetes Mellitus and Obesity." Diabetes Metab Syndr Obes. 2014; 7: 587-591.

Catol, AF. "Metabolic Mechanisms in Obesity and Type 2 Diabetes: Insights from Bariatric/Metabolic Surgery." Obes Facts. 2015; 8: 350-363.

Yang, Q. "Added Sugar Intake and Cardiovascular Diseases Mortality Among US Adults." JAMA Intern Med. 2014; 174(4): 516-524.

Klein, S. "Importance of Blood Glucose Concentration in Regulating Lipolysis During Fasting in Humans." Am J Physiol. 1990 Jan; 258(1 pt 1): E32-9.

Asif, M "The Prevention and Control the Type 2 Diabetes by Changing lifestyle and Dietary Pattern." J Educ Health Promot. 2014; 3:1.

Ley, SH. "Prevention and Management of Type 2 Diabetes: Dietary Components and Nutritional Strategies." Lancet. 2014 Jun 7; 383(9933): 1999-2007.

Evert, AB. "Nutrition Therapy Recommendations for the Management of Adults with Diabetes." Diabetes Care. 2013 Nov; 36(11): 3821-3842.

Gerich JE. "The Importance of Tight Glycemic Control." Am J Med. 2005 Sep; 118(Sppl 9a): 7S-11S.

Moodahadu, LS. "Tight Glycemic Control and Cardiovascular Effects in Type 2 Diabetic Patients." Heart Views. 2014 Oct-Dec; 15(4): 111-120.

Schelhase, KG. "Glycemic Control and the Risk of Multiple Microvascular Diabetic Complications." Fam Med. 2005; 37(2): 125-130.

Perreault, L. "Effect of Regression from Prediabetes to Normal Glucose Regulation on Long-Term Reduction in Diabetes Risk:

Results from the Diabetes Prevention Program Outcomes Study." Lancet. 2012 Jun; 379(9833): 2243-2251.

Malek, M. "Risk of Cancer in Diabetes". ISRN Endocrinol. 2013; 2013: 636927.

Harada, PHN. "Lipoprotein Insulin Resistance Score and Risk of Incident Diabetes During Extended Follow –Up of 20 Years: The Women's Health Study." J Clin Lipidol. 2017 Sep-Oct; 11(5): 1257-1267.

Obesity

Ofei, F. "Obesity-A Preventable Disease." Ghana med J. 2005 Sep; 39(3): 98-101.

Mitchell, N. "Obesity: Overview of an Epidemic." Psychtr Clin North Am. 2011 Dex; 34(4): 717-732.

Hruby, A. "The Epidemiology of Obesity: A Big Picture." Pharmacodynamics 2015 Jul; 33(7): 673-689.

Scherer, P. "Adipose Tissue". Diabetes. 2006 Jun; 55(6): 1537-1545.

Bray, GA. "Medical Consequences of Obesity." J Clin Endocrinol Metab. 2004 Jun; 89(6): 2583-2589.

Stapleton, PAS. "Obesity and Vascular Dysfunction." Pathophysiology. 2008 Aug; 1592); 79-89.

Matson, KL. "Treatment of Obesity in Children and Adolescents." J Pediatr Pharmacol Ther. 2012 Jan-Mar; 17(1): 45-57.

Yao, L. "Roles of the Chemokine System in Development of Obesity, Insulin Resistance, and Cardiovascular Disease." J Immun Res. 2014 (2014), article ID 181450, 11 pages.

Nuttall, FQ. "Body Mass Index-Obesity, BMI, and Health: A Critical Review." Nutr Today. 2015 May; 50(3): 117-128.

[177]

Balasan, GA. "Relationship Between Adiponectin, Obesity and Insulin Resistance." Rev Assoc Med Bras. 2015 jan-Feb; 61(1).

Chandran, M. "Adiponectin: More Than Just Another Fat Cell Hormone." Diabetes Care. 2003 Aug; 26(8): 2442-2450.

Paracchini, V. "Genetics of Leptin and Obesity: A Huge Review." Am J Epidemiology. 2005 Jul; 162(2): 101-114.

Kersten, S. "Mechanisms of Nutritional and Hormonal Regulation of Lipogenesis." EMBO Rep. 2001 Apr 15 2(4): 282-286.

Ruopeng, A. "Prevalence and Trends of Adult Obesity in the US, 1999-2012." ISRN Obesity. 2014, Article ID 185132, 6 pages, 2014.

Bose, M. "Stress and Obesity: The Role of the Hypothalmic-Pituitary-Adrenal Axis in Metabolic Disease." Curr Opin Endocrinol Diabetes Obes. 2009 Oct.\; 16(5): 340-346.

Hamdy, O. "Metabolic Obesity: The Paradox Between Visceral and Subcutaneous Fat." Curr Diabetes Rev. 2006 Nov; 2(4): 367-373.

Shuster, A. "The Clinical Importance of Visceral Adiposity: A Critical Review of Methods for Visceral Adipose Tissue Analysis." R J Radiol. 2012 Jan; 85(1009): 1-10.

Matsuzawa, Y. "Pathophysiology and Pathogenesis of Visceral Fat Obesity." Obes Res. 1995 Sep; 3 Suppl 2: 187S-194S.

Hamilton, MT. "Too Little Exercise Too Much Sitting: Inactivity Physiology and the Need for New Recommendations on Sedentary Behavior". Curr Cardiovasc Risk Rep. 2008 Jul; 2(4): 292-298.

Heart Disease

Cassar, A. "Chronic Coronary Artery Disease: Diagnosis and Management." Mayo Clin Proc. 2009 Dec; 84(12): 1130-1146.

Sigurdsson, AF. "What is the Real Cause of Heart Disease?" Doc's Opinion. June 3, 2012.

Alie, N. "Inflammation, Atherosclerosis, and Coronary Artery Disease: PET/CT for the Evaluation of Atherosclerosis and Inflammation." Clin Med Insights Cardiol. 2014; 8(Suppl 3): 13-21.

Shrivastava, AK. "C-Reactive Protein, Inflammation and Coronary Heart Disease." Egyptian Heart J. 2015 Jun; 67(2): 89-97.

Libby, P. "Inflammation and Cardiovascular Disease Mechanisms." Am J Clin Nutr. 2006 Feb; 83(2): 456S-460S.

Pries, AR. "Perspectives: Microcirculation in Hypertension and Cardiovascular Disease." Ur Heart J Suppl. 2014 Jan; 16(Suppl A): A28-29.

Mayet , J. "Cardiac and Vascular Pathophysiology in Hypertension." Heart. 2003 Sep; 89(9): 1104-1109.

Ridker, PM. "Anti-Inflammatory Therapies for Cardiovascular Disease." Eur heart J. 2014 Jul; 35(27): 1782-1791.

Pashkow, FJ. "Oxidative Stress and Inflammation in Heart Disease: Do Antioxidant Have Role in Treatment and/or Prevention?" Int J Inflammation. 2011(20111), article ID 514623, 9 pages.

Yang, Q. "Added Sugar intake and Cardiovascular Diseases Mortality Among US Adults." JAMA Intern Med. 2014; 174(4): 516-524.

Kearns, CE. "Sugar Industry and Coronary Heart Disease Research: A Historical Analysis of Internal Documents." JAMA Intern Med. 2016; 176911): 1680-1685.

Temple NJ. "Fat, Sugar, Whole Grains and Heart Disease: 50 Years of Confusion." Nutrients. 2016 Jan; 4(10). Pii:E39.

[179]

Klein, S. "Heart Disease: 17 Celebrities with Heart Problems." Huff Post Healthy Living. February 7, 2012.

Ertl G. "Healing After Myocardial Infarction." Cardiovasc Res. 2005 Apr. 1;66(10: 22-32.

Campbell TC. "The China Study: The Most Comprehensive of Nutrition Ever Conducted and the Startling Implications for Diet, Weight loss, and Long-term Health." May 11, 2006.

Esselstyn CB. "Prevent and Reverse Heart Disease: The Revolutionary, Scientifically Proven, Nutrition-Based Cure." January 31, 2008.

Hyman, M. " Blood Sugar Solution: The UltraHealthy Program for losing weight, Preventing Disease, and Feeling Great Now!" February 28, 2012.

Shabestari, AA. "Coronary Artery Calcium Score: A Review." Iran Red Crescent Med J. 2013 Dec; 15(12): e16616.

Shah, NR. "An Evidence-Based Guide for Coronary Calcium Scoring in Asymptomatic Patients without Coronary Heart Disease." Tex Heart Inst J. 2012; 39(2): 240-242.

Coyan, GN. "Diet and Exercise Interventions Following Coronary Artery Bypass Graft Surgery: A Review and Call to Action." Phys Sportsmed. 2014 May; 42(2): 119-129.

Poplin, R. "Prediction of Cardiovascular Risk Factors from Retinal Fundus Photographs via Deep Learning." Nature Biomed Engineer. 2018; 2: 158-164.

Stroke

Strandgaard, S. "Pathophysiology of Stroke." J Cardiovasc Pharmacol. 1990; 15(Suppl 1): S38-42.

World Health Organization. "The top 10 Causes of Death." WHO.Intghomortality.

Xing, Changhong. "Pathophysiologic Cascades in Ischemic Stroke." Int J Stroke. 2012 Jul; 7(5): 378-385.

Kollmar, R. "Ischemic Stroke: Acute Management, intensive Care, and future perspectives." Br J Anaesthesia. 2007 Jul; 99(1): 95-101.

Lakhan, SE. "Inflammatory Mechanisms in Ischemic Stroke: Therapeutic Approaches." J Transl Med. 2009; 7: 97.

Slark, J. "Risk Awareness in Secondary Stroke Prevention: A Review of the Literature." JRSM Cardiovasc Dis. 2014 Jan-Dec; 3: 204800401351437.

Khare, S. "Risk factors of Transient Ischemic Attack: An Overview." J Midlife Health. 2016 an-Mar; 7(1): 2-7.

Sorenson, AG. "Transient Ischemic Attack Definition, Diagnosis, and Risk Stratification." Neuroimaging Clin N Am. 20111 May; 21(2): 303-313.

Wu, CM. "Early Risk of Stroke After Transient Ischemic Attack." Arch Intern Med. 2007; 167(22): 2417-2422.

Saleem, M. "Role of Carotid Duplex Imaging in Carotid Screening Programs-An Overview." Cardiovasc Ultrasound. 2008; 6: 34.

Byrnes, KR. "The Current Role of Carotid Duplex Ultrasonography in the Management of carotid Atherosclerosis: Foundations and Advances." Int J Vasc Med. 2012 (2012), Article ID 187872, 10m Pages.

Wall, HK. "Addressing Stroke Signs and Symptoms Through Public Education: The Stroke Heroes Act FAST Campaign." Prev Chronic Dis. 2008 Apr; 5(2): A49.

Jin, J. "Warning Signs of a Stroke". JAMA. 2014; 311(16): 1704.

[181]

Forughi, M. "Stroke and Nutrition: A Review of Studies." Int J Med. 2013 May; 4(Suppl 2): S165-179.

Medeiros, F. "How Can Diet Influence the Risk of Stroke?" Int J Hyperten. 2012(2012), Article ID 763507, 7 pages.

Sarikaya, H. "Stroke Prevention-Medical and Lifestyle Measures." Eur Neurol. 20155; 73: 150-157.

Metabolic Syndrome

Kaur, J. "A Comprehensive Review on Metabolic Syndrome." Cardiol Res Prat. 2014; 204:943162.

Grundy, SM. "Obesity, Metabolic Syndrome, and Cardiovascular Disease." J Clin Endocrin Metab. 2004 Jun; 89(6): 2595-2600.

Kaplan, NM. "The Deadly Quartet. Upper Body Obesity, Glucose Intolerance, Hypertriglyceridemia, and Hypertension." Arch Intern Med. 1989; 149; 1514-1520.

Liu, L. "Impact of Metabolic Syndrome on the Risk of Cardiovascular Disease Mortality in the United States and Japan." AM J Cardiol. 2014, Jan; 113(1): 84-89.

Hutcheson, R. "The Metabolic Syndrome, Oxidative Stress, Environment, and Cardiovascular Disease: The Greatest Exploration." Exp Diabetes Res. 2012, Article ID 271028, 13 Pages.

Cabre, JJ. "Metabolic Syndrome as a Cardiovascular Disease Risk Factor: Patients Evaluated in Primary Care." BMC Public Health. 2008; 8:251.

Roberts, CK. "Metabolic Syndrome and Insulin Resistance: Underlying Causes and Modification by Exercise Training." Compr Physiol. 2103 Jan; 3(1): 1-58.

Saely, CH. "The Metabolic Syndrome, Insulin Resistance, and Cardiovascular Risk in Diabetic and Nondiabetic Patients." J Clin Endocrinol Metab. 2005 Oct; 90(10): 5698-5703.

Jouyandeh, Z. "Metabolic Syndrome and Menopause." J Diabetes Metab Disord. 2013; 12:1.

Marjani, A. "The Metabolic Syndrome Among Postmenopausal Women in Gorgan." Int J Endocrinol. 2012; 2012, Article ID 953627, 6 pages.

Gurka, MJ. "Progression of Metabolic Syndrome Severity During the Menopausal Transition." JAHA. 2016; 5:e003609.

Kim, HM. "The Effect of Menopause on the Metabolic Syndrome Among Korean Women." Diabetes Care. 2007 Mar; 30(3): 701-706.

Manzato, E. "Metabolic Syndrome and Cardiovascular Disease in the Elderly: The (Pro. V.A.) Study." Aging Clin Exp Res. 2008 Feb; 20(1): 47-52.

Daubenmieer, J. "Mindfulness Intervention for Stress Eating to Reduce Cortisol and Abdominal Fat Among Overweight and Obese Women: An Exploratory Randomized Controlled Stud." J Obes. 2011; 2011: 651936.

Guo, S. "Decoding Insulin Resistance and Metabolic Syndrome for Promising Therapeutic Intervention." J Endocrinol. 2014 Feb; 220: E1- 3.

Song, S. "Carbohydrate Intake and Refined-Grain Consumption are Associated with Metabolic Syndrome in the Korean Adult Population." J Acad Nutr Diet. 2014 Jan; 14(1): 54-62.

Schulze, MB. "Dietary Approaches to Prevent the Metabolic Syndrome: Quality Versus Quantity of Carbohydrates." Diabetes Care. 2004 Feb; 27(2): 613-614.

Qin, B. "Cinnamon: Potential Role in the Prevention of Insulin Resistance, Metabolic Syndrome, and Type 2 Diabetes." J Diabetes Sci Technol. 2010 May; 4(3): 685-93.

Fujioka, K. "The Effects of Grapefruit on Weight and Insulin Resistance to the Metabolic Syndrome." J Medicinal Food. 2006 mar; 9(1): 49-54.

Alzheimer's Disease

Neurgroschi, J. "Alzheimer's Disease: Diagnosis and Treatment Across the Spectrum of Disease Severity." Mt Sinai J Med. 2011 Jul-Aug; 78(4): 596-612.

Swerdlow, RH. "Pathogenesis of Alzheimer's Disease." Clin interv Aging. 2007 Sep; 2(3): 347-359.

Defina, PA. "Alzheimer's Disease Clinical and Research Update for Health Care Practitioners." J Aging Res. 2013 (2013), Article 207178, 9 pages.

Murphy, MP. "Alzheimer's Disease and the beta-Amyloid Peptide." J Alzheimers Dis. 2010 Jan; 19(1): 311.

Zhang, F. "Neuroinflammation in Alzheimer's Disease." Neuropsychiatr Dis Treat. 2015 Jan 30; 11: 243-56.

Solomon, A. "Advances in the Prevention of Alzheimer's Disease and Dementia". J Intern Med. 2014 Mar; 275(3): 229-250.

Johnson, KA. "Brain Imaging in Alzheimer's Disease." Cold Spring Harb Perspect Med. 2012 Ap; 2(4): a006213.

Yiannopulou, K. "Current and Future Treatments for Alzheimer's Disease." Ther Adv Neurol Disord. 2013 Jan; 6(1): 19-33.

Prasansuklab, A. "Amyloidosis in Alzheimer's Disease: The Toxicity of Amyloid Beta Mechanism of its Accumulation and

Implications of Medicinal Plants for Therapy." Evid Based Complement Alternat Med. 2013; 2013: 413808.

Zhang, X. "Pathological Role of Hypoxia in Alzheimer's Disease." Exp Neurol. 2010 Jun; 223(2): 299-303.

Peers, C. "Hypoxia and Alzheimer's Disease." Essays Biochem. 2007; 43: 153-64.

Roher, AE. "Cerebral Blood Flow in Alzheimer's Disease." Vasc Health Risk Manag. 2012; 8: 599-611.

Postiglione, A. "Cerebral Blood Flow in Patients with Dementia of Alzheimer's Type." 1993 Feb; 5(1): 19-26.

Sweeney, MD. "The Role of Brain Vasculature in Neurodegenerative Disorders." Nat Neurosci. 2018 Oct; 21(10): 1318-1331.

De la Torre, JC. "Can Disturbed Brain Microcirculation Cause Alzheimer's Disease?" Neurol Res. 1993 Jun; 15(3): 146-53.

Huang, CW. "Cerebral Perfusion Insufficiency and Relationships with Cognitive Deficits in Alzheimer's Disease: A Multiparametric Neuroimaging Study." Scientific Reports. 2018; 8: 1541.

Sierra-Marcos, A. "Regional Cerebral Blood Flow in Mild Cognitive Impairment and Alzheimer's Disease Measured with Arterial Spin Labeling Magnetic Resonance Imaging." Int J Alzheimers Dis. 2017; 2017: 5479597.

Zhou, J. "Association between Stroke and Alzheimer's Disease: Systematic Review and Meta-Analysis." J Alzheimers Dis. 2015; 43(2): 479-89.

Cole, GM. "Inflammation and Alzheimer's Disease." Neurobiol Aging. 2000 May-Jun; 21(3): 383-421.

Wyss-Coray, T. "Inflammation in Alzheimer's Disease-A Brief Review of the Basic Science and Clinical literature". Cold Spring Harb Perspect Med. 2012 Jan; 2(1): e006346.

Meraz-Rios, MA. "Inflammatory Process in Alzheimer's Disease." Front Integr Neurosci. 13 August 2013.

Hansen, DV. "Microglia in Alzheimer's Disease." J Cell Biol. DOI: 10. 1083/jcb.201709069.

[9]Smith, JC Rao, SM. "Physical Activity Reduces Hippocampal Atrophy in Elders at Genetic risk for Alzheimer's Disease." Front Aging Neurosci. 2014 April 23; 6:61.

Bherer, L. "A Review of the Effects of Physical Activity and Exercise on Cognitive and Brain Functions in Older Adults." J Aging Res. 2013; 2013: 657508.

[10]Balsamo, S. "Effectiveness of Exercise on Cognitive Impairment and Alzheimer's Disease." Int J Gen Med. 20-13; 6: 387-391.

Cancer

Russell, Sabin. "Nixon's War on Cancer: Why it Mattered." Fred hutch. Hutch News. Sept 21, 2016.

Sudhakar, A. "History of Cancer, Ancient and Modern Treatment Methods." J Cancer Sci Ther. 2009 Dec 1; 1(2): 1-4.

Dancey, JE. "The Genetic Basis for Cancer Treatment Decisions." Science Direct. 2012 Feb; 148(3): 409-420.

American Cancer Society. "Cancer Facts and Figures 2017." American Cancer Society 2017.

Tomasetti, C. "Stem Cell Divisions, Somatic Mutations, Cancer Etiology, and Cancer Prevention." Science 2017 Mar; 355(6331: 1330-1334.

Loeb, Lawrence. "Multiple Mutations and Cancer." PNAS 2003 Feb; 100(3): 776-781.

Tomlinson, I. 'How Many Mutations in a Cancer?" Am J Pathol. 2002 Mar; 160(3): 755-758.

Bukhtoyarov, OV. "Pathogenesis of Cancer: Cancer Reparative Trap." J Cancer Therapy. 2015; 6(5), Article ID: 56146, 13 Pages.

Berger, NA. "Obesity and Cancer Pathogenesis." Ann NY Acad Sci. 2014 Apr; 1311: 57-76.

Warburg, O. "On the Origin of Cancer." Science. 1956 Feb 24; 123(319): 309-14.

Liberti, MV. "The Warburg Effect: How Does it Benefit Cancer Cell?" Trends Biochem Sci. 2018 Mar; 41(3): 21-218.

Zong, WX. "Mitochondria and Cancer." Mol Cell. 2016 Mar 3; 61(5): 667-676.

Porporato, PE. "Mitochondrial Metabolism and Cancer." Cell Research. 2018; 28: 265-280.

Cui, H. "Oxidative Stress, Mitochondrial Dysfunction, and Aging." J Signal Transduct. 2012; 2012: 646354.

Boland, ML. "Mitochondrial Dysfunction in Cancer'. Front Oncol. 2013; 3: 292.

Gaude, E. "Defects in Mitochondrial Metabolism and Cancer." Cancer Metb. 2014; 2(10).

Eales, KL. "Hypoxia and Metabolic Adaptation of Cancer Cells." Oncogenesis. 2016 Jan; 5(1); e190.

Adamaki, M. "Cancer and the Cellular Response to Hypoxia." Pediatr Therapeut. 2012. S1: 002. Doi: 10.4172/2161-0665, S1-002.

Cosse, JP. "Tumor Hypoxia Affects the Responsiveness of Cancer Cells to Chemotherapy and Promotes Cancer Progression." Anticancer Agents Med Chem. 2008 Oct; 8(7): 790-7.

Cui, J. Xu, Y. "Hypoxia and Miscoupling Between Reduced Energy Efficiency and Signaling to Cell Proliferation Drive Cancer to Grow Increasingly Faster." J Mol Cell Biol. 2012; DOI: 10. 1093/mcb/mjs017.

Vaupel, P. The Role of Hypoxia-Induced Factors in Tumor Progression." The Oncologist. 2004 Nov; 9(Suppl 5): 10-17.

Koonin, EV. "Is Evolution Darwinian or/and Lamarkian." Biol Direct. 2009; 4:42.

Vineis, P. "Cancer as an Evolutionary Process at the Cell Level: An Epidemiological Perspective." Carcinogenesis. 2003 Jan; 24(1): 1-6.

Strom, M. "Cancer Theorist Paul Davies to Speak on the Disease's Evolutionary History. The Sunday Morning Herald. 1 December 2015.

Vaapil, M. "Hypoxic Conditions Induce a Cancer-Like Phenotype in Human Breast Epithelial Cells." PLoS One; 7(9): e46543.

Krock, BL. "Hypoxia-Induced Angiogenesis: Good and Evil. " Genes and Cancer. 2011 Dec; 2(12): 1117-1133.

Vicente-Duenas, C. "The Role of Cellular Plasticity in Cancer Development." Curr Med chem. 2009; 16(28): 3676-85.

Flavahan, WA. "Epigenetic Plasticity and the Hallmark of Cancer." Science. 2017 Jul 21; 357(6348).

Duncan, EJ. "Epigenetics, Plasticity, and Evolution: How Do We Link Epigenetic Change to Phenotype?" J Exp Zool B Dev Evol. 2014 Jun; 322(4): 208-220.

[188]

Zhang, C. "Cancer May be a Pathway to Cell Survival Under Persistent Hypoxia and Elevated ROS: A Model for Solid-Cancer Initiation and Early Development." Int J Cancer. 2015 May 1; 136(9): 201-11.

Abollo-Jimenez, F. "The Dark Side of Cellular Plasticity: Stem Cells in Development and Cancer." Prof Stanley Shostak (Ed.), ISBN: 978-953-307-225-8, In Tech.

Rakoff-Nahoun, S. "Why Cancer and Inflammation?" Yale J Biol Med. 2006 Dec; 79(3-4): 123-130.

Coussens, LM. "Inflammation and Cancer." Nature. 2002 Dec.19; 420(69017): 860-867.

Jiang, Y. "A Sucrose-Enriched Diet Promotes Tumorigenesis in Mammary Gland in Part Through the 12-Lipooxygenase Pathway." Canc Res. 2016 Jan 1; 76(1): 24-29.

[11]Santisrteban, GA. "Glycemic Modulation of Tumor Tolerance in a Mouse Model of Breast Cancer." Biochem Biophys Res Commun. 1985 Nov 15; 132(3): 1174-9.

Ryu, TY. "Hyperglycemia as a Risk Factor for Cancer Progression." Diabetes Metab J. 2014 Oct; 38(5): 330-336.

Klement, RJ. "Is There a Role for Carbohydrate Restriction in the Treatment and Prevention of Cancer?" Nutr Metab. 2011; 8: 75.

Griffeth, LK. "Use of PET/CT Scanning in Cancer Patients: Technical and Practical Considerations." Proc(Bayl Univ Med Cent). 2005 Oct; 18(4): 321-330.

Wang, M. "Cancer Risk Among Patients with Type 2 Diabetes Mellitus: A Population-Base Prospective Study in China." Scientific Reports. 2015; 5, Article number 11503.

Giovannucci, E. "Diabetes and Cancer." Diabetes Care. 2010 Jul; 33(7): 1674-1685.

Dewhirst, MW. "Exercise Effects Tumor Growth and Drug Response in a Mouse Model of Breast Cancer." JNCI. 2015 May; 107(5): djv089.

Jones, LW. "Effect of Aerobic Exercise on Tumor Physiology in an Animal Model of Human Breast Cancer." J Appl Physiol. 2010 Apr; 108(4): 1021.

Terra, Rodrigo. "Effect of Exercise on the Immune System: Response, Adaptation and Cell Signaling." Rev Med Exporte. 2012 may/Jun; 18(3): 208-214.

Cormie, P. "The Impact of Exercise on Cancer Mortality, Recurrence, and Treatment-Related Adverse Effects." Epidemiol Rev. 2017 Jan; 39(1): 71-92.

Brown, JC. "Cancer, Physical Activity, and Exercise." Compr Physiol. 2012 Oct; 2(4): 2775-2809.

Meyerhardt, JA. "Impact of Physical Activity on Cancer Recurrence and Survival in Patients with Stage III Colon Cancer: Findings from CALGB 89803." J Clin Oncology. 2006; 24(22): 3535-3541.

Dimeo. F. "Exercise for Cancer Patients: A New Challenge in Sports Medicine". Br J Sports Med. 2000; 34(3).

Stefani, L. "Clinical Implementation of Exercise Guideline to Cancer Patients: Adaptation of ACSM's Guidelines for the Italian Model." J Funct Morph Kinesiol. 2017 Jan 13.

Dennett, AM. "Moderate-Intensity Exercise Reduces Fatigue and Improves Mobility in Cancer Survivors: A Systematic Review and Meta- Regression." J Physiotherapy. 2016 Apr; 62(2): 68-82.

Stepien, K. "Hyperbaric Oxygen as an Adjunctive Therapy in Treatments of Malignancies, Including Brain Tumours." Med Oncol. 2016; 33(9): 101.

Allen, BG. "Ketogenic Diets as an Adjuvant Cancer Therapy: History and Potential Mechanism." Redox Biol. 2014; 2: 963-970.

Khodadadi, S. "Tumor Cells Growth and Survival Time with the Ketogenic Diet in Animal Models: A Systematic Review." Int J Prev Med. 2017; 8: 35.

Zi, F. "Metformin and Cancer: An Existing Drug for Cancer Prevention and Therapy (review)." Nov 14, 2017. https://doi.org/10.3892/ol.2017.7412.

Chapter 5: Linking Aging to Our Circulation

<u>The Aging Process</u>

Tosato, M. "The Aging Process and Potential Interventions to Extend Life Expectancy." Clin Interv Aging. 2007 Sep; 2(3): 401-412.

Wilhelm, T. "Neuronal Inhibition of the Autophagy Nucleation Complex Extends Life Span in Post-Reproductive C. Elegans." Genes Develop. 7 September 2017.

Nigam, Y. "Physiological Changes Associated with Aging and Immobility." J Aging Res. 2012; 2012, Article ID 468469, 2 pages.

Passarino, G. "Human Longevity: Genetics or Lifestyle? It Takes Two to Tango." Immun Ageing. 2016; 13:12.

Tosato, M. "The Aging Process and Potential Interventions to Extend Life Expectancy." Clin Ingterv Aging. 2007 Sep; 2(3): 401-4123.

Jin, KL. "Modern Biological Theories of Aging." Aging Dis. 2010 Oct; 1(2): 72-74.

Peng, C. "Biology of Ageing and Role of Dietary Antioxidants." Biomed Res Int. 2014; (2014); Article ID 831841, 13 pages.

Park, KL. "The Role of Antioxidants in Combating the Aging Process." Inquiry J. 2009; 13.

Chronological Versus Biological Aging

[12]Levine, ME. "Modeling the Rate if Senescence: Can Estimated Biological Age Predict Mortality More Accurately than Chronological Age?" J Gerontol A Biol Sci. 2013 Jun; 68(6): 667-74.

Jylhava, J. "Biological Age Predictors." EBioMedicine. 2017 Jul; 21: 29-36.

Yoo, J. "Biological Age as a Useful Index to Predict Seventeen-Year Survival and Mortality in Koreans." BMC Geriatr. 2017; 17: 7.

Stephen, Y. "How Old Do You Feel? Role of Age Discrimination and Biological Aging in Subjective Age?" PLOS One. March 4, 2015.

Choi, NG. "Discrepancy Between Chronological Age and Felt Age Group Difference in Objective and Subjective Health as Correlates." J Aging Health. 2014 Apr; 26(3): 458-473.

[13]Kekich, D. "How Old Are You Now? What's Your Biological Age?" Institute for Ethics and Emerging Technologies. May 21, 2015.

Premature Aging

Silva, PA. "The Dunedin Multidisciplinary Health and Development Study: A 15 Year Longitudinal Study." Paediatr Perinat Epidemiol. 1990 Jan; 491): 76-107.

Poulton, R. "The Dunedin Multidisciplinary Health and Development Study: Overview of the First 40 Years, with an Eye to the Future." Soc Psychiatry Psychiatr Epidemiol. 2015; 50(5): 679-693.

Belsky, DW. "Quantification of Biological Aging in Young Adults." PNAS. 2015; 112(30): E4104-E4110.

Lara, J. "A Proposed Panel of Biomarkers of Healthy Ageing." BMC Med. 2015; 13:222.

Burkle, A. "MARK-AGE Biomarkers of Ageing". Mechanisms of Ageing and Development." 2015 Nov; 151: 2-12.

Nakamura, E. "A Method for Identifying Biomarkers of Aging and Constructing an Index of Biological Age in Humans?" J Gerontol. 2007 Oct; 62(10): 1096-1105.

Dubowitz, N. "Aging is Associated with Increased HbA1c Levels, Independently of Glucose Levels and Insulin Resistance, and also with Decreased HbA1c Diagnostic Specificity." Diabet Med. 2014 Aug; 321(8): 927-35.

Warming, L. "Changes in Bone Mineral Density with Age in Men and Women: A Longitudinal Study." Osteoporos Int. 2002; 13(2): 105-12.

Kalyani, RR. "Diabetes and Altered Glucose Metabolism with Aging." Endocrinol Metab Clin North Am. 2013 June; 42(2): 333-347.

Kolovou, G. "Ageing Mechanisms and Associated Lipid Changes." Curr Vasc Pharmacol. 2014; 12(5): 682-9.

Pinto, E. "Blood Pressure and Ageing." Postgrtad Med J. 2007 Feb; 83(976): 109-114.

Blue Zone

Buettner, D. "The Blue Zone: Lessons for Living Longer From the People Who've Lived the Longest." Mass Market Paperback. October 19, 2010.

National Geographic. "5 "Blue Zones" Where the World's Healthiest People Live." National Geographic. April 6, 2017.

Singularity Hub Staff. "Blue Zones-Places in the World Where People Live and Stay Healthy." SingularityHub. July 20, 2009.

Bingham, K. "The Blue Zones: Lessons for Living Longer from the People." Blue Zone Study Guide. 2012.

Sisson, M. "7 Characteristics with Long Life (and How to Cultivate Them)." Mark's Daily Apple. May 15, 2013.

Atmon, G. "Genetics, Lifestyle and Longevity: Lessons from Centenarians." Appl Transl Genomics. 2015 Mar; 4: 23-32.

Myagi, S. "Longevity and Diet in Okinawa, Japan: Past, Present, and Future". Asia Pac J Public Health. 2003; 15 Suppl: S3-9.

Le Couteur, DG. "New Horizons: Dietary Protein, Ageing and the Okinawan Ratio." Age and Ageing. 2016 Jul; 45(4): 443-447.

Macvean, M. "Why Loma Linda Residents Live Longer than the Rest of Us: They Treat the Body Like a Temple." Los Angeles Times. Jul 11, 2015.

Research on Aging

Belluz, J. "Google is Super Secretive About its Anti-Aging Research. No One Knows Why." Vox. Apr 28, 2017.

Ruby, JG. "Estimates of the Heritability of Human Longevity are Substantially Inflated Due to Assortative Mating." Genetics. Nov 2018; 210(3): 1109-1124.

Gierman, H. "Whole-Genome Sequencing of the World's Oldest People." PLOS one. 2014 Nov; 9(11): e112430.

Williams, M. "Who Wants to Live Forever?: The Palo Alto Longevity Prize." HeroX.com.

Ferrucci, L. "The Baltimore Longitudinal Study of Aging (BLSA): A 50-Year-Long Journey and Plans for the Future." J Gerontology: Series . 2008 Dec; 63(12): 1416-1419.

National Institute of Aging. "BLSA's IDEAL Future."

Kirkland, S. "The Canadian Longitudinal Study on Aging: Study Design and Methods." Innovations in Aging. https://doi.org/10.1093/geroni/igx004.2641.

Wilcox, DC. "They Really are That Old: A Centenarian Prevalence in Okinawa." J Gerontology: Series A, 2008 Apr; 63(4): 338-349.

Bernstein, AM. "First Autopsy of an Okinawan Centenarian: Absence of Many Age-Related Disease." J Gerontology: Series A, 2004 Nov; 59(11): 1195-1199.

Pal, S. "Epigenetics and Aging." Sci Adv. 2016 Jul; 2(7): e1600584.

Sen, P. "Epigenetic Mechanisms of Longevity and Aging." DOI: https://doi.org/10.1016/j.cell.2016.07.050.

Aging Blood Vessels

Fye, WB. "William Osler." Clin Cardiol. 1988 May; 11(5): 356-358.

Bliss, M. "William Osler: A Life in Medicine." (2007). New York: Oxford University Press.

Fleg, JL. "Age-Associated Changes in Cardiovascular Structure and Function: A Fertile Milieu for Future Disease." Heart Fail Rev. 2012 Sep; 17(0): 545-554.

O'Rourke, MF. "Mechanical Factors in Arterial Aging: A Clinical Perspective". J Am Coll Cardiol. 2007 Jul; 50(1): 1-13.

Jani, B. "Ageing and Vascular Ageing". Postgrad Med J. 2006 Jun; 82(968): 357-362.

Mulligan-Kehoe, MJ. "Vasa Vasorum in Normal and Diseased Arteries". Circulation. 2014; 129: 2557-2566.

Lahteenvuo, J. "Effects of Aging on Angiogenesis." Circ Res. 2012 Apr 27; 110(9): 1252-64.

Groen, BB. "Skeletal Muscle Capillary Density and Microvascular Function Are Compromised with Aging and Type 2 Diabetes." J Appl Physiol. 2014 Apr; 116(8): 998-1005.

Kano, Yutaka. "Effect of Aging on the Relationship Between Capillary Supply and Muscle Fiber Size." Advances in Aging Res. 2013; 2(1): 37-42.

Edelberg, JM. "Aging and Angiogenesis." Front Biosci. 2003 Sep; 8: s1199-209.

Torregrossa, Ashley. "Nitric Oxide and Geriatrics: Implications in Diagnostics and Treatment of the Elderly." J Geriatr Cardiol. 2011 Dec; 8(4): 230-242.

Debbabi, H. "Increased Skin Capillary Density in Treated Essential Hypertensive Patients." Am J Hypertens. 2006 May; 19(5): 477-483.

Conese, M. "The Fountain of Youth: A Tale of Parabiosis, Stem Cells, and Rejuvenation." Open Med (Wars). 2017; 12: 376-383.

Katsimpardi, L. "Vascular and Neurogenic Rejuvenation of the Aging Mouse Brain by Young Systemic Factors." Science. 2014 may 9; 344(6184): 630-634.

Scudellari, M. "Ageing Research: Blood to Blood." Nature. 52015 Jan; 517: 426-429.

Eggel, A. "Parabiosis for the Study of Age-Related Chronic Disease." Swiss Med Wkly. 2014;144: w13914.

Gresham, GA. "Response of Vessels to Ischaemia." Eye. 1991; 5(Pt 4): 438-9.

Ferreira, JP. "Intima-Media Thickness is Linearly and Continuously Associated with Systolic Blood Pressure in a Population-Based Cohort (STANISLAS Cohort Study)." J Am Heart Assoc. 2016 Jun; 5(6).

Xu, J. "Vasa Vasorum in Atherosclerosis and Clinical Significance." Int J Sci. 2015 May; 16(5): 11574-11608.

Jarvilehto, M. "Vasa Vasorum Hypoxia: Initiation of Atherosclerosis." Science Direct. 2009 Jul; 73(1): 40-41.

Rittman, EL. "The Dynamic Vasa Vasorum." Cardiovasc res. 2007; 75: 649-658.

Jarvilehto, M. "Vasa Vasorum Hypoxia in Atherosclerosis obliterans, Peripheral Artery Disease and restless Leg Syndrome." OA Med Hypothesis. 2014 Jan; 2(1).

Kwon, TG. "The Vasa Vasorum in Atherosclerosis." J Am Coll Cardiol. 2015 Jun; 65(23).

Durham, AL. "Role of Smooth Muscle Cells in Vascular Calcification: Implication in Atherosclerosis and Arterial Stiffness." Cardioasc Res. 2018 Mar; 114(4): 590-600.

Chistiakov, DA. "Vascular Smooth Muscle Cell in Atherosclerosis." Acta Physiol. 2015 May; 214 (1): 33-50.

Muto, A. "Mechanisms of Vein Graft Adaptation to the Arterial Circulation: Insight into Neointimal Algorithm an Management Strategies." Circ J. 2010 Aug.; 74(8): 1501-12.

Zhang, H. "Artery Interposed to Vein Did Not Develop Atherosclerosis and Underwent Atrophic Remodeling in Cholesterol Fed Rabbits." Atherosclerosis. 2004 Nov; 177(1): 37-41.

Ranu, H. "Pulmonary Function Tests." Ulster Med J. 2011 May; 80(2): 84-90.

Torpy, JM. "Cardiac Stress Testing." JAMA. 2008; 300(15): 1836.

Heslop, CL. "Myeloperoxidase and C-Reactive Protein Have Combined Utility for Long-Term Prediction of Cardiovascular Mortality after Coronary Angiography." J Coll Cardiol. 2010 Mar; 55(11): 1102-9.

Oygarden, H. "Carotid Intima-Media Thickness and Prediction of Cardiovascular Disease." JAMA. 2017; 6: e0053313.

McQuilkin, GL. "Digital Thermal Monitoring (DTM) of Vascular Reactivity Closely Correlates with Doppler Flow Velocity." Conf Proc IEEE Eng Med Biol Soc. 2009; 2009: 1100-1103.

Pereira, T. "Novel Methods for Pulse Wave Velocity Measurement." J Med Biol Eng. 2015; 35(5): 555-565.

Chapter 6: Unleashing the Power of Our Circulation

Eat Right

Manzel, A. "Role of "Western Diet" in Inflammatory Autoimmune Diseases." Curr Allergy Asthma Rep. 2014 Jan; 14(1): 404.

Cordain, L. "Origins and Evolution of the Western Diet: Health Implications for the 21st Century." Am j Clin Nutr. 2005 Feb; 81(2): 341-354.

Romangnolo, D. "Mediterranean Diet and Prevention of Chronic Diseases." Nutrition Today. 2017 Sep/Oct; 52(5): 208-222.

Donahue RP. "Physical Activity and Coronary Heart Disease in Middle-aged and Elderly Men: Honolulu Heart Program." Am J Public Health. 1988 June: 78(6): 683-685.

Lohman, S. "A Brief History of Bread." 2012, Dec. History Stories. History.

Dernini, S. "Mediterranean Diet: From a Healthy Diet to a Sustainable Dietary Pattern." Front Nutr. 2015; 2: 15.

Mu, Q. "Leaky Gut as a Danger Signal for Autoimmune Diseases." Front Immunol. 2017; 8: 598.

Bischoff, SC. "Intestinal Permeability-A New Target for Disease Prevention and Therapy." BMC Gastroenterol. 2014; 14: 189.

Singh, RK. "Influence of Diet on the Gut Microbiome and Implications for Human Health." J Transl Med. 2017; 15: 73.

Hemarajata, P. "Effects of Probiotics on Gut Microbiota: Mechanisms of Intestinal Immunomodulation and Neuromodulation." Therap Adv Gastroenterol. 2013 Jan; 6(1): 39-51.

Washington State University. "Nutrition Basics." myNutrition. Washington State University.

Warne, RW. "The Micro and Macro of Nutrients Across Biological Scales." Intergr Comparat Biol. 2014 Nov; 54(5): 864-872.

Solon-Biet, SM. "Macronutrients and Calorie Intake in Health and Longevity." J Endocrinol. 2015 Jul; 226(1): R17-28.

Vergnaud, A-C. "Macronutrient Composition of the Diet and Prospective Weight Change in Participants of the Epic-Panacea Study." PLoS ONE. 8(3): e57300.

Group, E. "What Are Macronutrients?" Global Healing Center. 2017 May.

Shenkin, A. "Micronutrients in Health and Disease." Postgrad Med J. 2006 Sep; 82(971): 559-567.

PhysiciansCommittee. "Carbohydrates: Complex vs Simple Carbs." PCRM.com.

van Baak, MA. "Starches, Sugars and Obesity." Nutrients. 2011 Mar; 3(3): 341-369.

Ferretti, F. "Simple vs. Complex Carbohydrate Dietary Patterns and the Global Overweight and Obesity Pandemic." Int J Environ Res Public Health. 2017 Oct; 14(10): 1174.

Hartel, K. "Simple vs. Complex Carbohydrates." Fitday.com.

Wong, JM. "Carbohydrate Digestibility and Metabolic Effects." J Nutr. 2007 Nov; 137(11): 2539S-2546S.

Liu, AG. "A Healthy Approach to Dietary Fats: Understanding the Science and Taking Action to Reduce Consumer Confusion." Nutr J. 2017; 16: 53.

Lawrence, GD. "Dietary Fats and Health: Dietary Recommendations in the Context of Scientific Evidence." Adv Nutr. 2013 May; 4(3): 294-302.

Dinicolantonio, JJ. "The Cardiometabolic Consequences of Replacing Saturated Fats with Carbohydrates or Omega-6 Polyunsaturated Fats: Do the Dietary Guidelines Have it Wrong?" Open Heart. 2014; 1. doi: 10.1136/openhrt-2013-000032.

Siri-Tarino, PW. "Saturated Fats Versus Polyunsaturated Fats Versus Carbohydrates for Cardiovascular Disease Prevention and Treatment." Annu Rev Nutr. 2015; 35: 517-543.

Veum, VL. Dankel, SN. "Visceral Adiposity and Metabolic Syndrome After Very High-Fat and Low-Fat Isocaloric Diets: A Randomized Controlled Trial." Am J Clin Nutr. 2017 Jan; 105(1): 85-99.

Maholtra, A. "Saturated Fat Does Not Clog the Arteries: Coronary Heart Disease is a Chronic Inflammatory Condition, the Risk of

Which Can be Effectively Reduced from Healthy Lifestyle Interventions." Br j Sports Med. 2017 Apr; 51: 15.

Chowdhury R. "Association of Dietary Circulating, and Supplement Fatty Acids with Coronary Risk: A Systematic Review and Meta-Analysis." Ann Intern Med. 2014; 160(6): 398-406.

DiNicolantonio, JJ. "The Evidence for Saturated Fat and for Sugar Related to Coronary Heart Disease." Prog Cardiovasc Dis. 2016 Mar-Apr; 58(5): 464-472.

Jacobs, DR. "Food Synergy: An Operational Concept for Understanding Nutrition." Am J Clin Nutr. 2009 May; 89(5): 1543S-1548s.

Tapsell, L. "Foods and Food Components in the Mediterranean Diet: Supporting Overall Effects." BMC Med. 2014; 12: 100.

Hoffmann, I. "Transcending Reductionism in Nutrition Research." Am J Clin Nutr. 2003 Sep; 78(3): 514S-516S.

Fardet, A. "From Reductionist to a Holistic Approach in Preventive Nutrition to Define New and More Ethical Paradigms." Healthcare (Basel). 2015 Dec; 3(4): 1054-1063.

de Lorgeril, M. "Mediterranean Diet, Traditional Risk Factors, and the Rate of Cardiovascular Complications After Myocardial Infarction: Final Report of the Lyon Diet Hear Study." Circulation. 1999 Feb 16; 99(6): 779-85.

Eat Less

Rupp, R. "Clean Your Plate: Getting a Handle on Food Waste." National Geographic. March 31, 2015.

Wansink, B. "Consequences of Belonging to the "Clean Plate Club"." Arch Pediatr Adolesc Med. 2008 Oct; 162(10): 994-5.

Rubaum-Keller, I. "Hara Hachi Bu: Eat Until You are 80% Full." Huffpost the blog. Sep 21, 2011.

Mattison, JA. "Calorie Restriction Improves Health and Survival of Rhesus Monkeys." Nature Communications. 2017; 8, Article Number: 14063.

Weindruch, R. "Calorie Restriction and Aging." Sci Am. 1996 Jan; 274(1): 46-52.

Wahlberg, D. "Monkeys That Eat Less Live longer After All, University of Wisconsin Study Finds." Madison.com. Jan 18, 2017.

Colman, RJ. "Caloric Restriction Reduces Age-Related and All-Cause Mortality in Rhesus Monkeys." Nature Communications. 2014; 5, Article Number: 3557.

Trepanowski, JF. "Impact of Caloric and Dietary Restriction Regimens on Markers of Health and Longevity in Humans and Animals: A Summary of Available Finding." Nutr J. 2011; 10:107.

Collier, R. "Intermittent Fasting: The Science of Going Without,." CMAJ. 2013 Jun 11; 185(9): E363-E364.

Patterson, RE. "Intermittent Fasting and Human Metabolic Health." J Acad Nutr Diet. 2015 Aug; 115(8): 1203-1212.

Moro, T. "Effects of eight Weeks of Time-restricted Feeding (16/8) on Basal Metabolism, Maximal Strength, Body Composition, Inflammation, and Cardiovascular Risk Factors in Resistance-Trained Males." J Transl Med. 2016; 14: 290.

Longo, VD. "Fasting, Circadian Rhythms, and Time Restricted Feeding in Healthy Lifespan." Cell Metab. 2016 Jun 14; 23(6): 1048-1059.

Chaix, AS. "Time-Restricted Feeding is a Preventive and Therapeutic Intervention Against Diverse Nutritional Challenges." Cell Metab. 2014 Dec 2; 20(6): 991-1005.

Move More

Boughouts, LB. "Exercise and Insulin Sensitivity: A Review". Int J Sports Med. 2000 Jan; 21(1): 1-12.

Ivy, JL. "Muscle Glycogen Synthesis Before and After Exercise." Sports Med. 1991 Jan; 11(1): 6-19.

Jensen, TE. "Regulation of Glucose and Glycogen Metabolism During and After Exercise." J Physiol. 2012 Mar 1; 590(Pt 5): 1069-1076.

Adams, OP. "The Impact of Brief High-Intensity Exercise on Blood Glucose Levels." Diabetes Metab Syndr Obes. 2013; 6: 113-122.

Colberg, SR. "Exercise and Type 2 Diabetes." Diabetes Care. 2010 Dec; 33(12): e147-e167.

Way, KL. "The Effect of Regular Exercise on Insulin Sensitivity in Type 2 Diabetes Mellitus: A Systematic Review and Meta-Analysis." Diabetes Metab J. 2016 Aug; 40(4): 253-271.

Mul, JD. "Exercise and Regulation of Carbohydrate Metabolism." Prog Mol Biol Transl Sci. 2015 Aug; 135: 17-37.

Ross, R. "Does Exercise Without Weight Loss Improve Insulin Sensitivity?" Diabetes Care. 2003 Mar; 26(3): 944-945.

Trewin, AJ. "Exercise and Mitochondrial Dynamics: Keeping in Shape with ROS and AMPK." Antioxidants (Basel). 2018 Jan; 7(1): 7.

Richter, EA. "AMPK and the Biochemistry of Exercise: Implications for Human Health and Disease." Biochem J. 2009 Mar 1; 418(2): 261-275.

Petersen, AM. "The Anti-Inflammatory Effect of Exercise." J Appl Physiol. 2005 Apr; 98(4): 1154-62.

Beavers, KM. "Effect of Exercise Training on Chronic Inflammation." Clin Chim Acta. 2010 Jun 3; 411(0): 785-793.

Gleeson, M. "The Anti-Inflammatory Effects of Exercise: Mechanisms and Implications for the Prevention and Treatment of Disease." Nature Rev Immunology. 2011 Aug 5; 11(9): 607-15.

Hong, S. "Benefits of Physical Fitness Against Inflammation in Obesity: Role of Beta Adrenergic Receptors." Brain Behav Immun. 2014 Jul; 39: 113-120.

Heinonen, J. "Organ-Specific Physiological Responses to Acute Physical Exercise and Long-Term Training in Humans." Physiology (Bethesda). 2014 Nov; 29(6): 421-36.

Laughlin, MH. "Mechanisms for Exercise Training Induced Increases in Skeletal Muscle Blood Flow Capacity: Differences with Interval Sprint Training Versus Aerobic Endurance Training." J Physiol Pharmacol. 2008 Dec; 59(Suppl 7): 71-88.

Pereira, F. "Interval and Continuous Exercise Training Produce Similar Increases in Skeletal Muscle and Left Ventricle Microvascular Density in Rats." BioMed Res intern. 2013; Article ID 752817, 7 Pages.

Karimian, J. "Effect of Resistance Training on Capillary Density Around Slow and Fast Twitch Muscle Fibers in Diabetic and Normal Rats." Asian J Sports Med. 2015 Dec; 6(4); e24040.

Prior, SJ. "Increased Skeletal Muscle Capillarization After Aerobic Exercise Training and Weight Loss Improves Insulin Sensitivity in Adults with IGT." Diabetes Care. 2014 May; 37(5): 1469-1475.

Mcguire, BJ. "Estimation of Capillary Density in Human Skeletal Muscle Based on Maximal Oxygen Consumption Rates". Am J Physiol Heart Circ Physiol. 2003 Dec; 285(6): H2382-91.

Bloor, CM. "Angiogenesis During Exercise and Training". 2005 Dec; 8(3): 263-271.

Bruni, F. "The Ripped and the Righteous," New York Times. Jan 29, 2011.

Clear, J. "Learning from Superhumans: The Incredible Fitness and Success of Jack LaLanne." James Clear.

Be Better Informed

Mandela, N. "Brainy Quote".

Fleming, G. "What Are Core Academic Classes. And Why Are They Important?" Mar 17, 2017. ThoughtCo.

[14]Boswell, RG. "Food Cue Reactivity and Craving Predict Eating and Weight Gain: A Meta-Analytic Review." Obes Rev. 2016 Feb; 17(2): 159-77.

Kelly, B. "Television Food Advertising to Children: Global Perspective." Am J Public Health. 2010 Sep; 100(9): 1730-1736.

[15]Harris, JL. "Priming Effects of Televisions Food Advertising on Eating Behavior." Health Psychol. 2009 Jul; 238(4): 404-413.

Costa, SM. "Food Advertising and Television Exposure: Influence on Eating Behavior and Nutritional Status of Children and Adolescents." Arch Latinoam Nutr. 2012 Mar; 62(1): 53-9.

[16]Dietz, WH, Jr. "Do We Fatten Our children at the Television Set? Obesity and Television Viewing in Children and Adolescents". Pediatrics. 1985; 75: 807-12.

Mowery, YM. "A Primer on Medical Education in the United States Through the Lens of a Current Resident Physician." Ann Transl Med. 2015 Oct; 3(18): 270.

Duffy, TP. "The Flexner Report—100 Years Later." Yale J Biol Med, 2011 Sep; 84(3): 269-276.

Janik, E. "The Battle for Medicine's Soul: A Century of Alternative Remedies." Jan 19, 2014. Salon.com

Cancer Tutor. "How Flexner Report Hijacked Natural Medicine." Mar 11, 2017. Cancertutor.com.

Beck, AH. "The Flexner Report and the Standardization of American Medical Education." JAMA. 2004; 291(17): 2139-40.

Angell, M. "The Truth About the Drug Companies: How They Deceive Us and What to Do About It." (2005) New York: Random House Trade Paperbacks.

Weil, A. "Health and Healing: The Philosophy of Integrative Medicine." 2004. Houghton Mifflin Harcourt.

Weil, A. "What is Integrative Medicine." Weil: Andrew Weil, M.D. Drweil.com.

Frass, M. "Use and Acceptance of Complementary and Alternative Medicine Among the General Population and Medical Personnel: A Systematic Review." Ochsner J. 2012 Spring; 12(1): 45-56.

Tabish, SA. "Complementary and Alternative Healthcare: Is it Evidence-Based." Int J Health. 2008 Jan; 2(1): V-IX.

Ali, A. "Disease Prevention and Health promotion: How Integrative Medicine Fits." Am J Prevent Med. 2015 Nov; 49(5): S230240.

Metformin

[17]Barzilai, NR. "Targeting Aging with Metformin (TAME): A Study to Target Aging in Humans." Gerontol. 2016 Nov; 56(Suppl 3). Pages 199.

Nasri, H. "Metformin: Current Knowledge." J Res Med Sci. 2014 Jul; 19(7): 658-664.

Witters, LA. "The Blooming of the French Lilac." J Clin Invest. 2001 Oct; 108(8): 1105-1107.

Rojas, LBA. "Metformin: An Old But Still the Best Treatment for Type 2 Diabetes." Diabetology Metabol Synd. 2013; 5: 6.

Hostalek, U. "Therapeutic Use of Metformin in Prediabetes and Diabetes Prevention." Drugs. 2015; 75(10): 1071-1094.

Yanovski, JA. "Effects of Metformin on Body Weight and Body Composition in Obese Insulin-Resistant Children." Diabetes. 2011 Feb; 60(2): 477-485.

Bannister, CA. "Can People with Type 2 Diabetes Live Longer Than Those Without? A Comparison of Mortality in People Initiated with Metformin or Sulphonylurea Monotherapy and Matched, Non-Diabetic Controls." Diabetes Obes Metab. 2014 Nov; 16(11): 1165-73.

Martin-Montalvo, A. "Metformin Improves Healthspan and Lifespan in Mice." Nat Commun. 2013; 4: 23192.

Marycz, K. "Metformin Decreases Reactive Oxygen Species, Enhances Osteogenic Properties of Adipose-Derived Multipotent Mesenchymal Stem Cells in Vitro, and Increases Bone Density in Vivo." Oxida Med Cell Longev. 2016; 2016 Apr: 9785890.

Markowicz-Piasecka, M. "Metformin—A Future Therapy for Neurodegenerative Diseases." Pharma Research. 2017 December; 34(12): 2614-2627.

Goldberg, RB. "Effect of Long-Term Metformin and Lifestyle in the Diabetes Prevention Program and Its Outcome Study on Coronary Artery Calcium." Circ. 2017 Jul; 1361): 52-64.

Geerling, JJ. "Metformin Lowers Plasma Triglycerides by Promoting VLDL-Triglyceride Clearance by Brown Adipose Tissue in Mice." Diabetes. 2014 mar; 63(3): 880-91.

Eppinga, RN. "Effect of Metformin Treatment on Lipoprotein Subfractions in Non-Diabetic Patients with Acute Myocardial Infarction: A Glycometabolic Intervention as Adjunct to Primary coronary Intervention in ST Elevation Myocardial Infarction (GIPS-III) Trail." PLOS ONE. 11(1): e145719.

Wiernsperger, NF. "Microcirculation in Insulin Resistance and Diabetes: More Than Just a Complication". Diabetes Metab. 2003 Sep; 29(4 Pt2): 6S77-87.

Kasznicki, J. "Metformin in Prevention and Therapy." Ann Transl Med. 2014 Jun; 296): 57.

Suissa, S. "Metformin and Cancer: Mounting Evidence Against an Association." Diabetes Care. 2014 Jul; 37(7): 1786-1788.

Yin, M. "Metformin is Associated with Survival Benefit in Cancer Patients with Concurrent Type 2 Diabetes: A Systematic Review and Meta-Analysis." Oncologist. 2013; 18(12): 1248-1255.

[18]Coyle, C. "Metformin as an Adjuvant Treatment for Cancer: A Systematic Review and Meta-Analysis." Ann Oncol. 2016 Dec; 27(12): 2184-2195.

Dreyfuss, JH. "Metformin Significantly Reduces Risk of Many Cancers." April 17, 2016. MDalert.com

Hajjar, J. "Metformin: An Old Drug with New Potential." Exp Opin Invest Drugs. 2013; 22: 1511-1517.

Saftig, J. "Can a Diabetes Drug Prevent Cancer Death?" Life Extension Magazine. 2012 Feb. Lifeextension.com.

Wang, JC. "Suppression of Hypoxia-Induced Excessive Angiogenesis by Metformin Via Elevating Tumor Blood Perfusion." Oncotarget. 2017 Sep 26; 8(43): 73892-73904.

Beysel, S. "The Effects of Metformin in Type 1 Diabetes Mellitus." BMC Endoc Disord. 2018: 18: 1

Asif, M. "The Prevention and Control the Type-2 Diabetes by Changing Lifestyle and Dietary Pattern." J Educ Health Promot. 2014; 3:1.

Harsha, DW. "Weight Loss and Blood Pressure Control." Hypertension. 2008; 51: 1420-1425.

Davidson, JA. "Is Hyperglycemia a Causal Factor in Cardiovascular Disease." Diabetes care. 2009 Nov; 329(Suppl 2): S331-333.

O'Dea, K. "Marked Improvement in Carbohydrate and Lipid Metabolism in Diabetic Australian Aborigines After Temporary Reversion to Traditional Lifestyle." Diabetes. 1984 Jun; 33(6): 596-603.

Bio

Dr. Edmund Kwan was born in Seoul, South Korea. His family immigrated to America when he was nine years old. After graduating Georgetown Medical School, he completed a residency in general surgery followed by a plastic surgery residency at New York Presbyterian-Weill Cornell Medical Center. After an Aesthetic fellowship he has since been practicing reconstructive and cosmetic surgery in New York City. As a Clinical Professor of Surgery at New York Presbyterian Hospital, Dr. Kwan regularly teaches plastic surgery residents and students. Dr. Kwan volunteers on a medical missions team, travelling to South America and Africa annually for the past 10 years. His passion for healthy living and total body wellness has led him on a journey to teach, research and advise friends, family, patients, and the community.

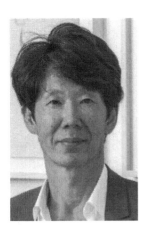

Made in the USA
Middletown, DE
04 July 2019